Decision Making in Palliative Care

by Peter Kaye

THIS BOOK IS DEDICATED TO
DAME CICELY SAUNDERS, OM
AN INSPIRATIONAL DOCTOR
AND TEACHER

CONTENTS

CONTENTS

CONTENTS

PREFACE

This book attempts to highlight some useful questions when dealing with common problems (both physical and psycho-social) in palliative care. It also explores how we make decisions, and how we can help patients to make decisions.

The Preview (on the next page), summarizes the ideas in the book. These ideas are discussed in more detail in the *Introduction*.

Simple flow-charts highlight some of the most important decisions. These charts are discussed in more detail in the section *How To Use The Charts*, after the Introduction.

I hope this book will provide a helpful starting point for newcomers to palliative care and perhaps offer some refreshment to the more experienced (in that "people need to be reminded more than they need to be instructed", as Dr Johnson once said).

Further reading is suggested at the end of the book, and includes any references mentioned in the text.

Abbreviations used in the text are explained at the end of the book.

I am very grateful to Linda Morrison for providing some stimulating conversations and ideas and to Kirsty Muirhead for carefully reading through the manuscript.

I would also like to thank the following for their helpful comments: Richard Abbatt, Peter Bailey, Phillip Ball, John Chambers, Christine Ellwell, Jenny Hedges, Barbara Malcomson, Jill Meredith, Angus Robinson, Hamish Ross, David Smart, John Smith, Ann Taylor-Chilton, Leslie Turner, Phillip Wiffin, Phil Wilkins, Mary Willows.

I am also grateful to Graham Watson for permission to reproduce his piece in the section on Carers, to my secretary Ann Bates for her patience in the face of my shortcomings, and to John Unwin and Hillary Austin for the expert typesetting.

PREVIEW

- **Medical decision-making** is complex and involves both facts and feelings. It is a science-using art that requires both judgement and communication skills (see box opposite). The American wit H L Mencken once said, "For every complex problem there is a simple solution – and it's usually wrong."

- **The flow-charts** in this book highlight important questions when making decisions in Palliative Care. They cover symptom control, psycho-social problems (eg, Anger, Denial) and management issues (eg Discharge planning). The charts are not evidence-based guidelines, they are simply a way of emphasising some important clinical decisions.

- **Some theoretical models** are described. The theories of Crisis intervention and Decision-making are particularly important..

- **The model called Crisis Intervention** underpins all the thinking in this book because its 4 styles of care, (support, counselling, explanation, problem-solving) relate to how decision-making takes place.

Patient's needs	Professional's role
Tolerate emotional distress	– Support
Adjust to emotional distress	– Counselling
Seek information	– Explanation
Consider options	– Problem-solving

- **Shared decision-making**, and the way it which has evolved over the past 40 years, is discussed in the section on Consultations. The theory is expanded here to encompass 2 essential aspects of palliative care: the team approach and the family.

- **Probability** has to be considered in most clinical decisions because the outcome is rarely certain (see Probabilities).

- **Patient's preferences** also affect decisions, which relate to attitudes, beliefs and personality (see Assumptions, Decision Analysis and Personality).

- **Medical decision-making** often happens in the context of stories (see Stories).

- **The Introduction** discusses these ideas in more detail.

Clinical decision-making is complex

A hospice doctor was asked to see a woman of 35 with breast cancer and brain metastases because she was complaining of shoulder pain. The brain metastases had caused a right-sided hemiplegia. The doctor examined her and decided that the aching pain in the right shoulder was probably due to the weakness around the shoulder joint. However, she also wanted to discuss her wish to die as soon as possible, her sense of rage at being so helpless and dependent on others, her frustration and fear that she had started having some difficulty in finding her words, and her disappointment that the recent brain irradiation had not improved her weakness. Her conversation with the doctor ranged back and forth between discussing analgesia for her shoulder pain, the effects of steroids, the chances of steroids improving her weakness, the likely course of her disease, her feeling unable to go on living like this, the effects of her illness on her young daughter, and the idea of having some sedation for a few days to help her cope with her emotional turmoil. Amidst all the questions (and the attempted answers) no clear consistent pattern emerged of her wishes. She hated taking medicines and wasn't sure what she really wanted. The doctor suggested she talk to her very supportive sister for a while and he would come back in a couple of hours. After an hour her sister approached the doctor with the results of their debate written on a piece of paper:

Tranquillizer\sedative?	–	YES
Increase in steroids?	–	NO
Painkiller for shoulder?	–	YES

This brief decision-making episode (one of many), illustrates that clinical decision-making often happens in a complex context of all sorts of tensions. After 48 hours she requested that the sedation be gradually reduced, and with the support of her family and the palliative care team she began to address the issues. A few days before she died, 3 weeks later, she even had a conversation with another patient to reassure her that dying was not distressing.

INTRODUCTION

> "Forget the scientific approach to clinical decision-making and you are a menace to your patients. Forget the human approach, and you ignore the aim of medicine"
>
> (Henrik Wulff)[1]

Life is complex. Every day we all have to make decisions. The American writer Bill Bryson (Notes from a small island) returning to the USA after living in England for many years commented on the difficulty of shopping when supermarkets offer such a vast range of products, such as 50 varieties of yoghurt! Too many decisions can be tiring and confusing.

Medical care is even more complex than supermarket shopping, and patients encountering scientific medicine can sometimes feel like a feather in the wind. Whether there is too little information, or too much, the problem is often that medical decisions involve uncertainty, and uncertainty is one of the most uncomfortable emotions to bear, and often leads to feelings of loss of control, frustration, fear and confusion.

When I first became a consultant I also felt confused at times. I slowly discovered that in some situations there were certain questions that could make my life a lot simpler (if I remembered to ask them). For example, some patients who came to the hospice wanted to discuss their past and future treatment in detail, and I discovered (eventually) that it was important to ask myself "Is the cancer histologically proven?" <u>before</u> discussing treatment decisions with the patient.

I realised that in complicated clinical situations there can be certain key questions that clarify decision-making. For example, should artificial hydration be given to a dying patient? The dilemma can provoke strong emotions and complex debates about rights, duties, quality of life, quality of death etc, but in practice the decision is often clarified by asking the simple key question:

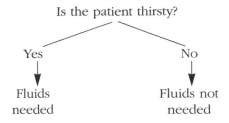

The flow-charts in this book try to identify some of the key questions that can help when making clinical decisions. The charts are the result of my own reading, my experiences and my sharing with colleagues, but they are only one person's perspective. Initially the charts were too complicated – so I re-designed them using a simple "yes" or "no" system (after all, even computers manage to work on a simple binary system). The charts are intended to be user-friendly, clear and simple.

There are different levels of decision-making that have to be considered: *internal* (which question to ask?), *clinical* (which drug to prescribe?), *inter-professional* (which team member is responsible?) and *organisational* (eg what equipment to buy?). All of these perspectives can arise in a given clinical situation, so each chart inevitably includes a mixture of these approaches, which is how it is in real-life.

The evidence is lacking for a lot of what we do, but most articles about evidence-based medicine emphasise the importance of starting by identifying the key clinical questions.[2.] Perhaps some of these charts will make a small contribution to the eventual development of clinical guidelines for particular problems.

The charts are NOT recommendations for "best practice" and they are not integrated care pathways (because a multi-disciplinary team did not write them). Such pathways will always be very difficult to produce because of variations in practice, the difficulties in getting research-based evidence, and the rapidly changing nature of medicine. And even when the best treatment has been proven, patients will still vary in their preferences for alternatives and outcomes. Care pathways will never entirely replace human judgement, because human interactions are so complex.

INTRODUCTION

Remarkably little is known about how doctors make decisions and it is a difficult area to study for at least 4 reasons:

- There is a wide variation in medical practice, suggesting doctors use different information (and possibly different attitudes) to make the same decisions.
- Studies have shown that doctors have difficulty recalling their decisions and providing rational reasons for their decisions.
- Many doctor-patient interactions occur in isolation and it is difficult to compare approaches.
- Studies (using actors) show that different doctors presented with an identical medical problem will make different decisions. Indeed the same doctor presented with an identical problem on separate occasions may make a different decision.

Traditionally doctor's decision-making and patient's decision-making have been quite separate. Medical decisions tend to be made by the medical team and the patient either consents or does not.

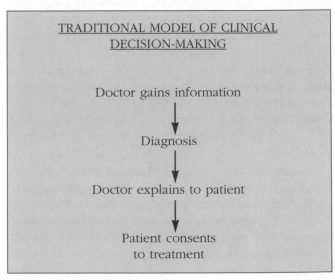

TRADITIONAL MODEL OF CLINICAL DECISION-MAKING

Doctor gains information

↓

Diagnosis

↓

Doctor explains to patient

↓

Patient consents
to treatment

This traditional model is based on the 2 key principles of making ethical medical decisions.
1 Will benefit outweigh harm?
2 Is it the patient's wish?

But this traditional model of decision-making is a "compliance model", because it is based on the notion of patient dependency. The patient simply agrees (or does not) to the decision that has been made. Informed consent – giving the patient both understandable information and time to reflect on its relevance to their own situation – is seen as important (and it is very important, and should not be ignored for reasons such as "the patient is too sick to understand", or "the research is so important and the risks are minimal" and only if the patient is unconscious or incompetent can it be waived[3]).

But in this traditional model the concept of "informed consent" is the only concession to the patient's perspective. The problem with the approach was neatly described in 1919 by the novelist Franz Kafka in his novel "A Country Doctor" (based on his favourite uncle Siegfried) when the doctor says "To write prescriptions is easy, but to come to an understanding with people is hard".[4]

The way clinical decisions get made has radically changed in the last 40 years, as summarised recently by Sir Cyril Chantler:

"Medicine used to be simple, ineffective and relatively safe. It is now complex, effective and potentially dangerous. The mystical authority of the doctor used to be essential for practice. Now we need to be open and work in partnership with our colleagues in health care and with our patients".

The latest version of the GMC's "Good medical practice" includes the responsibility to "respect the rights of patients to be fully involved in decisions about their care". But this idea is quite new. 30-40 years ago most doctors did not believe in sharing information or decisions with patients. Despite the calls of a few visionary doctors like Charles Fletcher[5] most doctors did not believe in sharing information with patients. When the TV programmes called "Your Life in Their Hands" came out in the 1960s, showing actual surgical operations, many doctors believed that disclosing such details was a "dangerous abuse" and the BMJ ran 4 articles about the dangers of giving patients too much information! A survey in 1968 showed that 88% of doctors did not always tell their patients the truth. But shared decision-making starts with the assumption that the truth is being openly told.

In 1993 a large study by both doctors and patients (who both examined videos of GP consultations) showed that shared decision-making is now considered to be an important part of any good medical consultation.[6]

A GOOD CONSULTATION

1. The doctor listens and looks interested
2. There is eye contact most of the time
3. The doctor explains (diagnosis\management)
4. The doctor allows time
5. The doctor is empathic, and does not trivialize the patients views and feelings
6. The doctor is warm and friendly (not abrupt or sarcastic)
7. The doctor is approachable\flexible (not authoritarian, judgmental or condescending).
8. The doctor is reassuring\encouraging\decisive (not indecisive or overconfident)
9. The doctor is relaxed
10. The patient is involved in decision-making

Cox and Mullholland, 1993

Shared decision-making is becoming a necessary method for the way decisions are made because more and more patients are wanting to be involved in decisions about their care, seeking advice not just from doctors but others as well. The idea of patient compliance is being replaced by that of "concordance" and of agreement and mutual responsibility for making decisions (I have tried to summarise how this idea of shared decision-making has evolved in the 2 sections on *Consultations*).

But one major difficulty with shared decision-making is the over-familiarity of professions with clinical decision-making, because they often under-estimate the complexity of the problem for patients (and this idea is discussed in more detail in the section on Thinking). Even a "simple" decision, like starting a new drug, often involves a lot of "invisible" information. Clinical experience provides a "fast-track" through the process, because we have done it so many times before, but some patients may want to understand the background logic and the background assumptions that are being made. How many potential questions arise whenever a drug is prescribed?

PRESCRIBING A DRUG – SOME QUESTIONS

Which drug is most appropriate?
Why is it preferred to others?
How does it act?
How do we know?
Has the patient tried it before?
- How long ago?
- How long for?
- Did it help?
- How often did the patient take it?
- Why was it stopped?
What chance does it have of helping?
What is the evidence?
Does the patient know anyone using it?
Does the patient have worries about this drug?
Does it have side-effects?
What are the probabilities of benefit/harm?
Will benefit outweigh harm?
Is the outcome uncertain?
Should the uncertainty be discussed?
Does the patient want to take it?
Will it interact with other drugs?
What form is preferred (eg liquid or tablet)?
Is swallowing difficult?
Which route will be best (oral, PR, SC etc)?
Who is in charge of the patient's medicines?
Do they understand what the drugs are for?
Do relevant others (eg family) disagree?
Do others need explanation?
How long will it be needed?
Who will monitor it?
What if it doesn't work?
When might it be stopped?
Who will decide?

INTRODUCTION

This book is full of theories, because no-one yet knows how medical decisions are made. If it was known how decisions were made there could be clear universal clinical guidelines for particular problems. Guidelines are coming[7] (see Guidelines) but they are difficult and expensive to produce, and very few guidelines are evidence-based (and indeed the evidence for most of what we do is still missing). So theories are inevitable, because a lot of the time they are all we have got.

Theories are very important. All thinking involves theories and assumptions. Facts are needed, of course, to make medical decisions. To quote Sir Theodore Fox (editor of the Lancet for 20 years), "Wherever a doctor meets a new patient or a new problem, he ought to have at his disposal every known fact that may help him". But we also need theories because facts alone are like a collection of bricks until we have a theory, to give them structure and purpose. A theory may change or develop over time, and may just be a story we are telling ourselves, but it remains essential. Albert Einstein the great scientific genius, once said "It is only theory that decides what we manage to observe" and the psychologist Kurt Lewin once wrote "There is nothing so practical as a good theory".

In a recent article in the British Medical Journal called "The importance of theories in health care". Priscilla Alderson wrote:

"Theories are at the heart of healthcare practice. All thinking involves theories. Theories range from explicit hypotheses to working models and frameworks of thinking about reality. Because theories powerfully influence how evidence is collected, analysed, understood, and used, it is practical and scientific to examine them. When theories are implicit *their power to clarify (or confuse) works unnoticed. It is important, scientifically and practically, to recognise implicit theories: they powerfully influence understandings of health care".*[8]

It is important to describe explicitly some of the implicit assumptions, or at least the ones that I can recognise, that underlie the theories in this book. Note that some of the assumptions might not be accepted by certain cultures. They include:

- Medical decisions flow through relationships. The spoken work is the most important tool in medicine.

- Our personal prejudices often remain invisible to us.

- If health-care professionals use clumsy language it can cause pain.

- Patients are frequently dissatisfied with doctor's communication skills.

- Family dynamics can have a powerful effect on a patient's decisions.

- Medical decisions are most likely to be effective if they are seen as occurring in the context of complex, interacting (and changing) social, emotional and spiritual factors.

- Clinical decisions are more effective when there is good communication between professionals.

- It is best for patients who are facing serious progressive illness to stand half way between hope and hopelessness (see *Attitudes*).

- It is best for patients to be aware of their own dying and for families to communicate openly about dying.

A theory of decision-making, like all psychological theories, has to be built on the 3 inter-related aspects of being: thinking, feeling and acting.[9] There has been a century of debate among psychologists about which comes first, thoughts or feelings. In fact they are intimately inter-related. In his excellent book "How the mind works" Steven Pinker writes: *"Intelligence is the pursuit of goals in the face of obstacles Since we cannot pursue all our goals at once we have to match our goals to the best time to achieve them. Emotions are therefore related to thinking, and are mechanisms that help us to prioritise our goals".*[10] Emotions are also related to posture and preparation for movement, and therefore to behaviour.

The theory of decision-making (set out in the section called *Decision-making I*) is based on the same 3 elements: tolerating emotional distress, finding and evaluating the best available information and selecting the best course of action by comparing options.

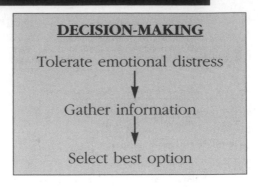

DECISION-MAKING

Tolerate emotional distress

↓

Gather information

↓

Select best option

Time is needed for important decisions, to discuss with others, to evolve new perspectives and to resolve emotional distress. The importance of time is often overlooked, and important decisions may have to evolve over a period of time. The Hippocratic teachings emphasised the importance of spending several days just observing and talking with patients, before trying to make the right decisions.

Emotional distress in the patient (anxiety, anger, exhaustion) can block decision-making. Rational argument cannot overcome muddled thinking that is due to an emotional reaction, and sometimes the emotions have to be dealt with first. This is discussed in more detail in the section called *Crisis Intervention*.

But emotions may not simply block the process, they may affect the decisions that get made. Decision-making may not be a one-off rational event but a dynamic situation transformed by the current emotions of the deciders. Emotions can affect decision-making in various ways: distress in the doctor or nurse who is giving advice, or family disagreements, or transference (wanting to please a doctor), or fear of criticism (eg from colleagues), or lack of trust (in doctors or information) or a recent traumatic experience (eg related to a similar decision) can all powerfully influence decision-making.

Emotional regression to a childlike state is quite common in physical illness. Often it is temporary, but sometimes it is part of a dependent personality, preferring others to take responsibility ("Mother has decided that she is not going to make any more decisions"). This is discussed further in the section on *Transactional Analysis*.

To make informed decisions we need information
How can we be sure we are using the most accurate information? Medicine is a knowledge-based activity, and the knowledge base is currently doubling every 19 years. There are now over 22,000 medical journals (with over 3700 on Medline). Reports of original research are far too numerous to be of practical use. The only way to cope with the information overload is to concentrate on review articles. The Cochrane collaboration is now doing this, and prepares up-to-date reviews of randomised controlled trials[11] (see *Appendix II*). The NHS information Authority was established in October 1998 to develop electronic records (with 24 hour instant access to patient information) and a National Electronic Library for health information (available to the public, patients, clinicians and managers) – the NHS Net. This will hopefully ensure that doctors and patients are better informed and better able to share in decisions.[12]

In an article called "What clinical information do doctors need?"[13], Richard Smith, editor of the BMJ, concluded "The doctor's information tool of the future might be some sort of combination between the patient record and the Internet, with the doctor and the patient positioned together at the intersection but not having to pay attention to the technology. Probably there will be no single tool but a family of tools, and I suspect that whatever sophisticated tools may be developed, the major source of information will remain colleagues". Meanwhile, we have to consider how to find the best information and how to explain it (see *Explanation* and *Information*).

Comparing options is the final step in decision making, and involves imagining the outcomes of the various options. Ways of doing this, or helping patients to do it, are discussed in the sections on Problem Solving and in Decision-making II. But in medical care, outcomes are often uncertain or based on probabilities. Clinical decisions often involve risk. As the American wit Yoggi Berra said, "It is hard to make predictions, especially about the future". All decisions happen under 3 possible conditions: certainty, risk, and uncertainty. <u>Certainty</u> means there is a single known outcome of known probability. <u>Risk</u> means that there are various possible outcomes, each of which can be assigned a probability. <u>Uncertainty</u> means that the probabilities of various outcomes are unknown (although the outcomes themselves may be known). The way we communicate risk to patients is discussed in the section called *Probabilities*.

The ability to think is obviously necessary in order to make decisions. This can be a problem when patients are intermittently confused. Is the patient competent to make a decision? (see Ethical decisions). Whenever we make decisions, we take in information and assume that our basic inferences are logical – but are they? Logic is needed to interpret information. A logical deduction is when 2 premises lead up to and justify a conclusion, eg

Premise 1:   Dr Brown is on call on Tuesdays.
Premise 2:   It is Tuesday.
Conclusion: Therefore, Dr Brown is on call.

But in complex situations we often abandon logic in favour of rules of thumb, and patients do not always draw logical conclusions from the information.[14] The problem is that a premise can be seem true, but because it is incompletely true it can lead to a false conclusion, eg

Premise 1:   Radiotherapy is used to treat cancer.
Premise 2:   I have cancer.
Conclusion: Therefore, I should receive radiotherapy.

Professionals are also capable of making such mistakes, and our own logic can be suspect. In an article called "Listen to the patient" a doctor described how he and a patient were in disagreement about a particular course of action, and he wrote: "She was of course absolutely right. The patient had thought about it in ways much more rational and profound than I had".[15]

Patients' preferences also affect decisions, as well as statistical probabilities. For example imagine a patient deciding about chemotherapy. The decision to have a treatment that will cause severe side-effects will depend on both the probability that it will help and also on the patient's preferences.

Outcome	Probability	Strength of preference of patient
CURE	1%	++++++
NO CURE	99%	+

Decision analysis is a mathematical method for comparing probabilities and preferences, in order to choose a preferred course of action.[16] I was surprised to discover that there is a specific mathematical function ("expected utility") to measure the benefits of a particular decision. It has apparently been used in business for some years, and although it is, as yet, rarely used in clinical care it is used in health policy or when considering the best form of treatment for a particular disease. In fact a "science" of decision-making has been developing over the past 30 years in policy making, and draws on economics, management science, philosophy, psychology, social science and statistics as well as, in the case of medical policies, the clinical sciences.

Most people are poor statisticians. The brain can only process a limited amount of data, so we tend to use crude rules of thumb, eg we tend to believe that the more memorable the event, the more likely it is to recur. Another fallacy is that if a person or thing resembles a category in our own minds then we believe they are more likely to belong to that category.

The principle of decision analysis is simple. It separates out the components of a decision using a decision tree, then calculates the probability and preference for each component. Drawing a decision tree can be useful in

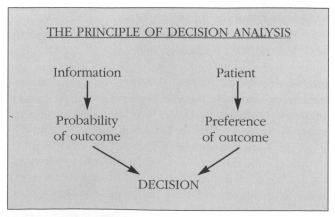

THE PRINCIPLE OF DECISION ANALYSIS

Information   Patient

Probability   Preference
of outcome   of outcome

DECISION

itself (even without the mathematics) when considering a large amount of information (see *Decision Analysis*).

It is easy to make incorrect assumptions about patients' preferences. Patients differ in their preferences (see *Personality*). For example a study of 87 patients with advanced lung cancer, who had all received cisplatin chemotherapy, showed that they had a wide variety of attitudes to chemotherapy.[17] Most patients said they would not choose chemotherapy even for a survival value of 3 months, unless it also controlled symptoms. But some patients said they would choose chemotherapy even for a survival benefit of as little as 1 week, whilst others said they would not choose it even for a survival benefit of 24 months. Some other examples of the variation in patients attitudes are discussed in the section called *Assumptions*.

Intuition is very important for decision-making. Research on 2000 patients with brain damage showed that people who consistently make poor decisions (eg about jobs or gambling) lack the ability to make unconscious use of memories of past emotions, rewards or punishments. (Science 1997; 275: 1269)

Intuition is at the opposite end of the spectrum to decision analysis. Intuition means making a decision based on feelings, and is necessary if the facts are not available. It involves a single global analysis of the whole problem. The advantage is that many complex preferences and beliefs can be incorporated into the decision.

But the disadvantage of using intuition is that it can make major simplifying assumptions, either because of the fallibility of human memory or because of stongly held, but incorrect, beliefs (see *Intuition*).

Judgement means making decisions based on indications when the facts are not certain (and may involve intuition). Professor Sir David Weatherall, the molecular biologist wrote in 1995 in his book Medicine and the Quiet Art – medical research and patient care: "Caring for sick people involves making considered judgements on the basis of limited evidence and information. At best, we are slowly reaching the stage at which we are aware of how little we know".[18] So most clinical decisions involve judgement. But what is happening when we make judgements? Can we improve our ability to make judgements? A very interesting book called "The Anatomy of Judgement" by Abercrombie examines in detail what happens when we make judgements, and concludes that even seeing or taking in information involves making internal judgements of which we are generally unaware. Becoming more aware of the internal influences on our judgements helps us to make better judgements, and the way to do this is to become more aware of the alternative judgements made by others. This is an important argument for discussing decisions with others as often as possible. "Discussion in a group does for thinking what testing on real objects does for seeing; we can see our assumptions and some other ways of thinking" [19] (see *Judgement*).

Story-telling is unavoidable during a consultation. Illness calls for stories.[20] Illness is almost always an important landmark in the whole story of a person's life.[21] Stories have a powerful influence on decision-making. The way the patient recounts their story affects the decisions that are made, and the way the story is shortened into a "medical history" and passed on from professional to professional also affects decisions (see *Stories*).

Most people relate to stories better than to statistics. TV soap operas and medical dramas can have a powerful influence on patient's decisions about their own health care. Clinicians sometimes communicate risks and benefits to patients in terms of stories about other patients. If a doctor wants to reassure or convince a patient about a some medical fact or opinion there is no better way than saying "A patient of mine had a similar condition to you and had the treatment and did very well". This can be very persuasive, but should not replace a factual explanation of risks and benefits, where possible.

Words and stories not only describe reality, but they also contribute to that reality[22] (which is why telling children they are naughty can become a self-fulfilling prophecy!). One role of the palliative care professional can be facilitating an alternative story (a "joint narrative") that makes sense of the situation from the patient's point of view.[23] The experience of meeting a doctor or nurse becomes part of the patient's story and part of the influence on their decisions ("the doctor was so kind, that I decided to go in to the hospice after all").

Allowing the patient space to tell their story, and to control the introduction of topics into the conversation can increase the diagnostic information available to the doctor.[24] A mutually developed dialogue, in which the patient does not have to be deferential to the doctor is more satisfactory to both parties and also more effective in the task of shared decision-making. (This is discussed further in the section on *Leadership*).

In conclusion, decision-making is at the heart of medical care. Improving our decision-making skills, and our understanding of how patients make decisions, will improve the quality of our care.

References

1 Henrik Wulff. Lancet 1988; 351: 1070

2 Rosenberg W, Donald A. Evidence-based medicine: an approach to clinical problem-solving. BMJ 1995; 310: 1122–6

3 Smith R. Informed consent: the intricacies. BMJ 1998; 314: 1059–60

4 Kafka F. Wedding preparations in the country and other stories. Harmonsworth: Penguin, 1982:119

5 Smith T. Charles Fletcher at 80: Happy Birthday – and sorry. BMJ 1991; 303: 6

6 Cox J, Mullholland H. An instrument for assessment of video-tapes of GP performances. BMJ 1993; 306: 1202-3

7 Fletcher SW, Fletcher RH. Development of clinical guidelines. Lancet 1998; 352: 1876

8 Alderson P. The importance of theories in healthcare. BMJ 1998; 317: 1007-10

9 Freeling P, Gask L. Sticks and stones. BMJ 1988; 317: 1028-9

10 Pinker S. How the Mind Works 1997. Allen Lane, the Penguin Press

11 Chalmers I. The Cochrane collaboration: Preparing, maintaining and disseminating systematic reviews of the effects of health care. Ann N. Y. Acad Sci 1993; 703: 156–163

12 Wyatt J, Keen J. The NHS's new information strategy. BMJ 1998; 317: 900

13 Smith R. What information do doctors need? BMJ 1996; 313: 1062-8

14 Tomassi P. Logic and Medicine in Phillips CI (Ed) Logic and Medicine 1995 BMJ Publishing Group

15 Macbeth Pitkin R. Listen to the patient. BMJ 1998; 316: 1252

16 Thornton JG, Lilford RJ, Johnson N. Decision analysis in medicine. BMJ 1992; 304: 1099-103

17 Silvestri G, Pritchard R, Gilbert Welch H. Preferences for chemotherapy in patients with advanced non-small cell lung cancer: descriptive study based on scripted interviews. BMJ 1998; 317: 771-5

18 Weatherall D. Medicine and the Quiet Art – medical research and patient care. 1995 Oxford University Press

19 Abercrombie MLJ. The anatomy of judgement. An investigation into the process of perception and reasoning. 1960. Free Association Books, London 1989

20 Greenhalgh T, Hurwitz B, Why study narrative? BMJ 1999; 318: 48-50

21 Brody H. My story is broken; can you help me fix it? Medical ethics and the joint construction of narrative. Lit Med 1994; 13: 79-92

22 Seale C. Theories and studying the care of dying people. BMJ 1988; 317: 1518-2

23 Hudson Jones A. Literature and medicine: narrative ethics. Lancet 1997; 349: 1243-6

24 Ainsworth-Vaughn N. Claiming power in Doctor–Patient Talk. 1998 New York: Oxford University Press

HOW TO USE THE CHARTS

The charts in this book are meant to be a simple tool for highlighting important questions and decisions. I have tried to put the questions in roughly the order they may be considered in a clinical case. They are NOT meant to be authoritarian, logical steps – they are merely ideas about useful clinical questions in the form of a chart.

In making the charts I have tried to identify some KEY questions which can help when making clinical decisions.

I have tried to keep the flow charts as simple as possible. The basic framework I have tried to use is:

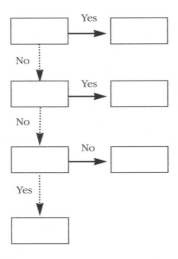

Clinical decision-making is highly complex (as discussed briefly in the introduction) and these charts are NOT meant to be complete statements on how to manage each problem.

In other words, these simple charts are NOT formal clinical guidelines. (Nor are they clinical protocols, classification trees, clinical algorithms or integrated care pathways.) Ideal clinical guidelines (or integrated care pathways) would have the following characteristics:

- evidence based
- derived from expert opinion
- each response predicting the next question

- every possible outcome considered
- modified by clinical experience
- based on decision analysis
- quantitative weighting of each outcome
- evaluated on real patients.

Very few such protocols exist (and they are proving very difficult to develop, even for simple clinical decisions) These charts are not intended to be clinical guidelines but simply a way of highlighting important clinical decisions.

The notes provide further discussion of some of the most important clinical questions and decisions.

I hope that the charts and notes will also be useful for teaching, by providing the basis for a mini-tutorial on each subject.

ANAEMIA

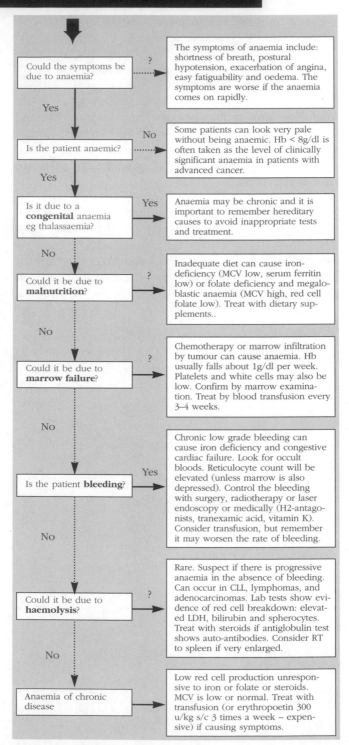

Could the symptoms be due to anaemia? **?**

The symptoms of anaemia include: shortness of breath, postural hypotension, exacerbation of angina, easy fatiguability and oedema. The symptoms are worse if the anaemia comes on rapidly.

Yes

Is the patient anaemic? **No**

Some patients can look very pale without being anaemic. Hb < 8g/dl is often taken as the level of clinically significant anaemia in patients with advanced cancer.

Yes

Is it due to a **congenital** anaemia eg thalassaemia? **Yes**

Anaemia may be chronic and it is important to remember hereditary causes to avoid inappropriate tests and treatment.

No

Could it be due to **malnutrition**? **?**

Inadequate diet can cause iron-deficiency (MCV low, serum ferritin low) or folate deficiency and megaloblastic anaemia (MCV high, red cell folate low). Treat with dietary supplements..

No

Could it be due to **marrow failure**? **?**

Chemotherapy or marrow infiltration by tumour can cause anaemia. Hb usually falls about 1g/dl per week. Platelets and white cells may also be low. Confirm by marrow examination. Treat by blood transfusion every 3–4 weeks.

No

Is the patient **bleeding**? **Yes**

Chronic low grade bleeding can cause iron deficiency and congestive cardiac failure. Look for occult bloods. Reticulocyte count will be elevated (unless marrow is also depressed). Control the bleeding with surgery, radiotherapy or laser endoscopy or medically (H2-antagonists, tranexamic acid, vitamin K). Consider transfusion, but remember it may worsen the rate of bleeding.

No

Could it be due to **haemolysis**? **?**

Rare. Suspect if there is progressive anaemia in the absence of bleeding. Can occur in CLL, lymphomas, and adenocarcinomas. Lab tests show evidence of red cell breakdown: elevated LDH, bilirubin and spherocytes. Treat with steroids if antiglobulin test shows auto-antibodies. Consider RT to spleen if very enlarged.

No

Anaemia of chronic disease

Low red cell production unresponsive to iron or folate or steroids. MCV is low or normal. Treat with transfusion (or erythropoetin 300 u/kg s/c 3 times a week – expensive) if causing symptoms.

ANAEMIA

Is it symptomatic?
Anaemia that has developed gradually may cause no symptoms even if the Hb level is below 8 g/dl. Don't assume that anaemia needs treating just because the haemoglobin level is low.

It is iron deficiency anaemia?
Microcytic hypochromic anaemia suggests iron deficiency which is usually due to chronic haemorrhage rather than malnutrition alone. Serum ferritin is low but total iron binding capacity is elevated (whereas in anaemia of chronic disease including carcinomas serum ferritin is elevated and iron-binding is low). Consider doing occult bloods to look for chronic haemorrhage. Oral iron elevates the haemoglobin 1g/dl per week.

Is the MCV increased?
Macrocytic anaemia (MCV above 96) suggests folate deficiency which may be dietary, if the patient has not had folate in the diet for 4-6 weeks. Patients with rapidly growing tumours or treatment with methotrexate are especially at risk. 5mg folate daily is adequate treatment. Remember that alcoholism and hepatic disease also increase the MCV.

Is it multi-factorial?
In advance disease many of these mechanisms are operating – dietary deficiencies, bleeding, anaemia of chronic disease, and rarely haemolysis.

Is blood transfusion indicated?
If the patient is still bleeding blood transfusion is not indicated since it will simply worsen the bleeding.

Has the patient had a blood transfusion before?
If a previous blood transfusion did not help then it usually not worth repeating but if a previous blood transfusion relieved symptoms then another blood transfusion is usually indicated. Each unit of packed red cells increases the haemoglobin by 1 g/dl. Aim for a post transfusion haemoglobin of 11 to 12 g/dl (eg a patient with Hb of 8 g/dl would normally be given 3 – 4 units).

How should blood be given?
Frusemide 20-40 mg with alternate units should be given to prevent fluid overload and heart failure. Each unit should be administered slowly over 4 to 6 hours and it is advisable to administer no more than 2 units per day. If a patient has had a previous transfusion reaction due to red cell antibodies (rhesus, kell etc) the lab needs to know.

What about erythropoietin?
Erythropoietin is very expensive at the moment and tends to be reserved for patients with anaemia secondary to chronic renal failure. It may come to have a place in some anaemias in palliative care practice.

See also: Bleeding

ANALGESICS 1 – USAGE

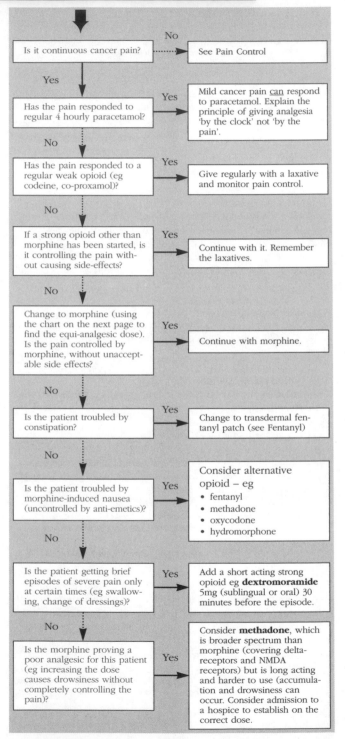

Is it continuous cancer pain?	No →	See Pain Control
Yes ↓		
Has the pain responded to regular 4 hourly paracetamol?	Yes →	Mild cancer pain <u>can</u> respond to paracetamol. Explain the principle of giving analgesia 'by the clock' not 'by the pain'.
No ↓		
Has the pain responded to a regular weak opioid (eg codeine, co-proxamol)?	Yes →	Give regularly with a laxative and monitor pain control.
No ↓		
If a strong opioid other than morphine has been started, is it controlling the pain without causing side-effects?	Yes →	Continue with it. Remember the laxatives.
No ↓		
Change to morphine (using the chart on the next page to find the equi-analgesic dose). Is the pain controlled by morphine, without unacceptable side effects?	Yes →	Continue with morphine.
No ↓		
Is the patient troubled by constipation?	Yes →	Change to transdermal fentanyl patch (see Fentanyl)
No ↓		
Is the patient troubled by morphine-induced nausea (uncontrolled by anti-emetics)?	Yes →	Consider alternative opioid – eg • fentanyl • methadone • oxycodone • hydromorphone
No ↓		
Is the patient getting brief episodes of severe pain only at certain times (eg swallowing, change of dressings)?	Yes →	Add a short acting strong opioid eg **dextromoramide** 5mg (sublingual or oral) 30 minutes before the episode.
No ↓		
Is the morphine proving a poor analgesic for this patient (eg increasing the dose causes drowsiness without completely controlling the pain)?	Yes →	Consider **methadone**, which is broader spectrum than morphine (covering delta-receptors and NMDA receptors) but is long acting and harder to use (accumulation and drowsiness can occur. Consider admission to a hospice to establish on the correct dose.

28

ANALGESICS 1 – USAGE

Is it a constant pain?
This section is about the use of analgesics for <u>constant</u> aching pain. (For intermittent pains, see Pain Control). If a patient is getting a constant aching pain they need regular analgesia. Teach them to take it "by the clock, not by the pain" and write out a drug card for them.

Has the patient already tried any analgesics?
The analgesic history can give you helpful clues about how to manage the pain. For example if the patient has tried taking two Solpadol tablets (which contains 30mg codeine plus 500mg paracetamol – like Tylex and Kapake) and noticed that the pain went for 2 hours and then returned, it guides you. It means that 60mg codeine is giving only 2 hours pain control, therefore the patient needs to start a stronger regular analgesic, eg morphine 5mg 4 hourly, or a 25mcg\hr fentanyl patch.

What is the "analgesic ladder"?
The analgesic ladder is simply a common-sense approach to choosing an appropriate analgesic for the severity of pain, eg:
• mild pain – paracetamol
• moderate pain – codeine
• severe pain – morphine or fentanyl

How do you select the right analgesic?
Pain is invisible so you have to be guided by the patient's description, plus the response to analgesics already tried, plus the patient's behaviour – eg a patient lying still and sweating and groaning with pain would be started on Diamorphine 2–5mg IM rather than parac-etamol.

Is morphine the best analgesic for severe cancer pain?
Morphine has been considered the best strong anal-gesic for continuous cancer pain with the advantages of a short half-life (2.5 hours) and no maximum dose, but other opioid analgesics can have advantages, eg:
• fentanyl – fewer side-effects
• methadone – broader spectrum and safe in renal failure
• dextromoramide – short-term boost in analgesia.

See also: Analgesics 2 – Doses

CHART FOR CHANGING ORAL ANALGESICS

(a guide to decide on the current dose)

			Morphine 4 hourly
Co-proxamol	2 tabs	≅	5mg
Codeine	60 mg	≅	5mg
Dihydrocodeine	60 mg	≅	5 mg
Pethidine (oral)	100 mg	≅	5 mg
Oxycodone (oral)	5 mg	≅	5 mg
Pentazocine	50 mg	≅	5 mg
Dipipanone	10 mg	≅	5 mg
Tramadol	50 mg	≅	7.5 mg
Methadone	see box below		
Buprenorphine	0.2 mg	≅	10 mg
Dextromoramide	5 mg	≅	10 mg
Phenazocine	5 mg	≅	25 mg
Hydromorphone	5 mg	≅	30 mg
Fentanyl Patch	25 mcg/hr	≅	5–15 mg

Note: oxycodone and hydromorphone are clinically very similar to morphine.

Example
A patient taking 0.4mg buprenorphine TDS would be given 20mg morphine 4 hourly for an equi-analgesic dose (and 30mg 4 hourly if not pain controlled).

Methadone
Methadone can be effective (especially in nerve pain) when morphine is not, but it is difficult to use. Consider admission to a hospice before starting it, because there is a danger of accumulation and sedation a few days after starting it. Low doses can be effective even if the morphine dose is high. One method is to add methadone 5–10mg BD and give 5–10mg PRN for any breakthrough pain then gradually reduce the morphine dose.

This table is about equi-analgesic doses of opioid analgesics. It is a clinical guide, for swapping <u>ORAL</u> analgesics, but it only applies to analgesics being taken regularly – it may not apply for single doses.

When do analgesics need to be changed?
The principle is to use an analgesic that works without causing unacceptable side-effects and which can be adjusted to suit the level of pain. It is sensible for the doctor to prescribe analgesics he or she has experience of using. Some analgesics have a high incidence of side-effects (eg pentazocine often causes dysphoria) and some have a ceiling dose, and are only effective at lower doses either because of a toxic metabolite (eg norpethidine) or because analgesic effect does not increase above a certain dose (eg buprenorphine). Some analgesics are useful in certain situations, eg the fentanyl patch is less constipating and useful in dysphagia or patients with renal failure or poor compliance, methadone is a broad spectrum analgesic (active at mu, delta and NMDA receptors), dextromoramide is useful to provide a brief boost to analgesia (eg before painful dressings).

Why are equi-analgesic doses so important?
It is important to know the approximate equivalent doses of analgesics when changing from one to the other. If the dose of the new analgesic is too strong the patient will feel drowsy, and may get other side-effects, (nausea, confusion, hallucinations) which will put them off taking it. Similarly if the dose of the new analgesic is too low, the pain will return, and again the patient may lose confidence in the new analgesic.

What about the half-life?
The half-life of these analgesics varies. Pain relief may last 2–3 hours (eg pethidine, dextromoramide) 4 hours (eg morphine) 6 hours (eg phenazocine) 8 hours (eg buprenorphine) or even 12 hours (eg methadone). The important point is that they are given <u>regularly</u>, to control the constant pain.

What is "opioid-rotation"?
Opioid "rotation" is better termed opioid substitution, and is considered (a): if there are unacceptable side-effects (eg changing morphine to fentanyl to reduce constipation) or (b): if the pain is a constant aching pain (ie the type that usually responds well to an opioid) and yet for some reason is responding poorly to the analgesic being used – for example methadone may control a constant pain that has not responded to morphine.

See also: Analgesics 1 – Usage

ANGER

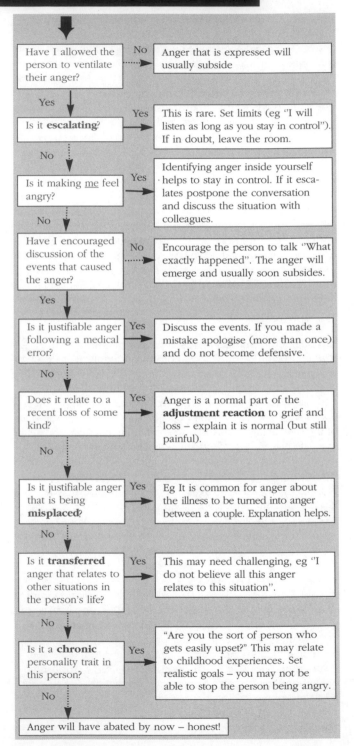

Have I allowed the person to ventilate their anger?	No →	Anger that is expressed will usually subside
↓ Yes		
Is it escalating?	Yes →	This is rare. Set limits (eg "I will listen as long as you stay in control"). If in doubt, leave the room.
↓ No		
Is it making me feel angry?	Yes →	Identifying anger inside yourself helps to stay in control. If it escalates postpone the conversation and discuss the situation with colleagues.
↓ No		
Have I encouraged discussion of the events that caused the anger?	No →	Encourage the person to talk "What exactly happened". The anger will emerge and usually soon subsides.
↓ Yes		
Is it justifiable anger following a medical error?	Yes →	Discuss the events. If you made a mistake apologise (more than once) and do not become defensive.
↓ No		
Does it relate to a recent loss of some kind?	Yes →	Anger is a normal part of the **adjustment reaction** to grief and loss – explain it is normal (but still painful).
↓ No		
Is it justifiable anger that is being misplaced?	Yes →	Eg It is common for anger about the illness to be turned into anger between a couple. Explanation helps.
↓ No		
Is it transferred anger that relates to other situations in the person's life?	Yes →	This may need challenging, eg "I do not believe all this anger relates to this situation".
↓ No		
Is it a chronic personality trait in this person?	Yes →	"Are you the sort of person who gets easily upset?" This may relate to childhood experiences. Set realistic goals – you may not be able to stop the person being angry.
↓ No		

Anger will have abated by now – honest!

What does anger mean?
Anger is a normal emotion, especially when confronted with a crisis (ie a temporary inability to cope with a change). It can be a compliment if a patient trusts you enough to get angry in your presence, and trusts your professionalism enough that it will not adversely affect their care.

Is the person angry?
Anger may be obvious, but it can be hidden or disguised – eg being withdrawn, being difficult, calling for frequent attention, failing to comply with previously-agreed treatments or sometimes "aggressive humour". For example a patient who laughed and joked all the time was challenged: "I appreciate your sense of humour but sometimes feel it hides other strong feelings" and this opened up an important conversation about his anger and various frustrations (financial as well as physical) and allowed the consultation to become more real.

Are you fearful of anger in patients or relatives?
It is very helpful to develop skill at handling anger appropriately. When anger occurs it often leads to a situation where important communications can happen, if it is handled correctly. If anger is directed at colleagues never criticise. Listen and empathise (eg "I can understand that would make you feel very angry").

Has the person had an opportunity to express their anger?
Anger that remains unexpressed often blocks decision-making or useful discussion. Give the person an opportunity to talk about the situations(s) that made them angry and to "ventilate" their feelings. It is better to ask "what happened?" (and the feelings will emerge) rather than "do you feel angry?" (since many people feel guilty or ashamed about their anger). Once anger is verbalised it tends to subside.

What is the cause of the anger?
It is only possible to make sense of anger <u>after</u> it has been ventilated ("like making tea <u>after</u> the kettle has boiled"). Analysing the anger can often lead to a useful discussion.

• Is it <u>long-standing</u> (personality problem)?

• Is it <u>normal</u> (adjustment to loss)?

• Is it <u>justified</u> (eg medical error)?

• Is it <u>misplaced</u> (eg projected onto wife)?

• Is it <u>transferred</u> (from elsewhere)?

Most families simply want information and an opportunity to express their feelings and worries.

ANXIETY

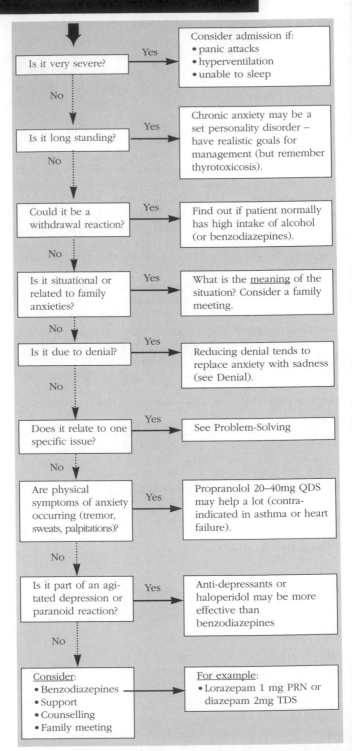

Is it very severe? — Yes → Consider admission if:
- panic attacks
- hyperventilation
- unable to sleep

No ↓

Is it long standing? — Yes → Chronic anxiety may be a set personality disorder – have realistic goals for management (but remember thyrotoxicosis).

No ↓

Could it be a withdrawal reaction? — Yes → Find out if patient normally has high intake of alcohol (or benzodiazepines).

No ↓

Is it situational or related to family anxieties? — Yes → What is the <u>meaning</u> of the situation? Consider a family meeting.

No ↓

Is it due to denial? — Yes → Reducing denial tends to replace anxiety with sadness (see Denial).

No ↓

Does it relate to one specific issue? — Yes → See Problem-Solving

No ↓

Are physical symptoms of anxiety occurring (tremor, sweats, palpitations)? — Yes → Propranolol 20–40mg QDS may help a lot (contra-indicated in asthma or heart failure).

No ↓

Is it part of an agitated depression or paranoid reaction? — Yes → Anti-depressants or haloperidol may be more effective than benzodiazepines

No ↓

<u>Consider:</u>
- Benzodiazepines
- Support
- Counselling
- Family meeting

→ <u>For example:</u>
- Lorazepam 1 mg PRN or diazepam 2mg TDS

Is it severe?
Severe anxiety can be extremely unpleasant and should be considered a medical emergency, if it is disturbing a patients sleep or especially if they are experiencing panic attacks or hyperventilation and tetany (tingling especially around the mouth due to metabolic alkalosis) consider admission.

Is it long-standing?
Chronic anxiety maybe part of a personality disorder and it maybe unrealistic to expect to reduce it. Remember to exclude thyrotoxicosis if the patients has been on Benzodiazepines long-term, do not stop them.

Is it alcohol-withdrawal?
Certain withdrawal of alcohol (or Benzodiazepines) can cause an anxiety state which can develop into paranoia and psychotic agitation. In far advanced disease sometimes the best management is to re-start a patient's regular alcohol intake.

Is it situational?
If there is a pattern to the anxiety and it only occurs in certain situations it can help to analyse the cause, and possibly to avoid it occurring in the future. Has the patient a history of anxiety in certain situations such as claustrophobia.

Is it related to a specific fear?
Sometimes a patient needs help deciding what is triggering the anxiety. A useful technique to explore the issue can be that of "tracking". Noting key words (or issues) during the patient's conversation and repeating them back to the patient (eg "Your daughter?") can sometimes lead to the real underlying issue.

Are the family anxious?
Sometimes treating the patient alone does not resolve the problem. If the family is anxious it triggers the patient's anxiety. Family anxiety and patient anxiety tend to become a vicious circle. Sometimes the best way forward is to hold a family meeting and to tackle the anxiety as a family problem, and a family pattern. This is almost always helpful in reducing anxiety levels (see Family Meetings).

ASCITES

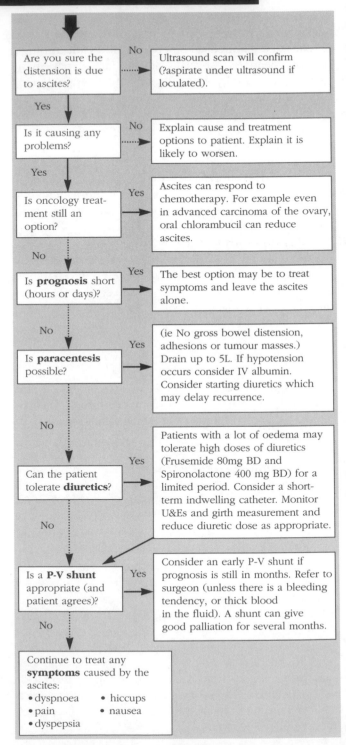

Are you sure the distension is due to ascites? → No → Ultrasound scan will confirm (?aspirate under ultrasound if loculated).

Yes ↓

Is it causing any problems? → No → Explain cause and treatment options to patient. Explain it is likely to worsen.

Yes ↓

Is oncology treatment still an option? → Yes → Ascites can respond to chemotherapy. For example even in advanced carcinoma of the ovary, oral chlorambucil can reduce ascites.

No ↓

Is prognosis short (hours or days)? → Yes → The best option may be to treat symptoms and leave the ascites alone.

No ↓

Is paracentesis possible? → Yes → (ie No gross bowel distension, adhesions or tumour masses.) Drain up to 5L. If hypotension occurs consider IV albumin. Consider starting diuretics which may delay recurrence.

No ↓

Can the patient tolerate diuretics? → Yes → Patients with a lot of oedema may tolerate high doses of diuretics (Frusemide 80mg BD and Spironolactone 400 mg BD) for a limited period. Consider a short-term indwelling catheter. Monitor U&Es and girth measurement and reduce diuretic dose as appropriate.

No ↓

Is a P-V shunt appropriate (and patient agrees)? → Yes → Consider an early P-V shunt if prognosis is still in months. Refer to surgeon (unless there is a bleeding tendency, or thick blood in the fluid). A shunt can give good palliation for several months.

No ↓

Continue to treat any **symptoms** caused by the ascites:
- dyspnoea
- pain
- dyspepsia
- hiccups
- nausea

Is the distension due to ascites (fluid)?

Abdominal distension may be due to tumour, bowel destruction, a very large liver or ascites (which simply means free fluid in the abdominal cavity). Free fluid causes the physical side of "shifting dullness". If in doubt, ultrasound scan is very helpful.

Is the ascites due to cancer?

In advance cancer abdominal ascites is almost always malignant, but it is worth remembering that there are other causes of ascites (cirrhosis, tuberculosis).

Has it been "tapped" before?

If the fluid has already been successfully drained by paracentesis it is usually an easy procedure to repeat the drainage if necessary. However it there is uncertainty that the abdominal distension is due to ascites (or whether the ascites is locculated), ultra sound scan should be considered before a first paracentesis.

Is it causing symptoms?

Symptoms include discomfort and difficulty bending, dyspnoea and gastric reflux (dyspepsia, hiccups, nausea). Secondary leg oedema can occur. One option may be to treat the secondary symptoms and leave the ascites alone, especially in a patient with a short prognosis.

Does the patient need urgent relief?

The quickest way of providing relief is parcentesis.

Can the patient tolerate high dose diuretics?

A combination of Frusimide 80mg daily and Spironolactone 200mg daily can slow down the recurrence of malignant ascites, especially after a paracentesis. This is useful treatment if the patient not only has ascites but also leg oedema. But the diuretics may cause unacceptable urinary frequency (and spironolactone can cause nausea.) If high dose diuretics are started monitor (U and E levels and abdominal girth measurements.) Reduce the dose once the ascites has resolved otherwise the patient can become dehydrated.

Is the fluid white and milky?

White milky fluid is called "chylous" and is due to a leak of lymphatic fluid from the thoracic duct, usually because it has been invaded by carcinoma. It is very difficult to manage, it tends to recur quickly after paracentesis and does not respond to diuretics, and the fluid is too thick usually to consider a PV shunt. Usually it is a pre-terminal event.

Does the patient need a shunt?

A peritoneo-venous shunt can be a very effective way of managing ascites, particularly in patients with a long prognosis (to avoid the need of repeated paracentesis.) A shunt can be inserted under local anaesthetic but is usually preferably done under general anaesthetic. It is contra-indicated if the patient is anti-coagulated or if the fluid is thick or blood stained fluid. A shunt can last many months. 30% of them eventually block and may need replacing.

ASSESSMENT

SETTING THE SCENE	ASSESSING THE PROBLEMS
⬇	⬇

SETTING THE SCENE

Do I have the medical notes? Do I need to have permission to see the patient?

Yes ⬇

Is this the right time and place for assessment? Am I the right person to do it?

Yes ⬇

Has the patient had the choice of being accompanied by a friend or relative?

Yes ⬇

Have I spent a few moments making 'social' contact?

Yes ⬇

Have I:
1. Introduced myself (name and role)?
2. Explained the purpose of this visit?
3. Set a time boundary?

Yes ⬇

Have I dealt with any over-riding medical priority, such as severe pain or vomiting?

Yes ⬇

Start full assessment (which may take more than one interview).

ASSESSING THE PROBLEMS

Have I asked for a narrative of medical events from the patient's point of view?

Yes ⬇

Have I enquired about symptoms and examined the patient?

Yes ⬇

Have I asked the patient what their **main CONCERNS** are at present?

Yes ⬇

Have I asked about their understanding of their illness, and their aims and expectations?

Yes ⬇

Have I drawn a family tree and asked what other family members understand about the illness?

Yes ⬇

Have I explained any changes to the medication, written a **DRUG CARD** and made a **PLAN** for the future?

Yes ⬇

Document decisions in the notes (? exclude confidential information).

Have I set the scene?

Setting the scene often gets forgotten but is essential preparation. Initial social contact is very important. Patients want and need to trust you. This is easier if they like you. This is more likely if you make a brief social contact with them in a friendly way before you do anything else.

Do I understand the patient's perspective?

A narrative by the patient is often helpful – eg it would help me to understand things from your point of view – how did it all start?" On the other hand patients can only tell their story so many times. If the patient has already seen many other professionals it may be best to get straight to the main concerns.

Have any symptoms been missed?

After discussing the main problems ask systematically about all symptoms (a check list in the notes helps).

Do I understand the patient's main concerns?

The role of the professional is to be a "midwife" for the patient's concerns. Ask about the patients "ICE" (which, like an iceberg, is usually nine tenths hidden).

I	= Ideas (Beliefs experiences)	– about the past
C	= Concerns (worries, difficulties)	– about the present
E	= Expectations (Aims, Hopes)	– about the future

Have I drawn a family tree?

A family tree is an essential part of the assessment (see Family Tree).

Have I written a drug card?

Explanation of medication using a written drug card makes a huge difference to care (see Prescribing).

Have I interlaced the conversation with questions about feelings

(eg "How do you feel about what we have discussed?" or "What did you feel then?").

Have I made a plan?

The ability to summarise the main problems and make a plan is an important characteristic of a professional. Making a plan involves the skill of shared decision-making.The plan should be transferable to different care settings.

Have you asked the patient?

Making shared decisions with patients who cannot speak or write can be very challenging. For example discussing the pros and cons of starting a PEG feeding gastrostomy for a patient who can only communicate with great difficulty can be very time-consuming – but it remains essential.

Ask the Patient

A man of 45 with multiple system atrophy and quadraplegia was unable to move or speak, and communicated by blinking. He was cared for by his wife with the help of the palliative care team. He developed severe dysphagia complicated by aspiration and a PEG was offered to him repeatedly. Feeding was slow and laborious (and exhausting) and became almost continuous but whenever PEG feeding was discussed and offered he declined.

Have you explained clearly enough?

When patients make decisions that seem illogical it can be important to explore their underlying assumptions. A woman with distressing and troublesome incontinence of urine repeatedly refused a catheter, for several weeks, until a doctor finally explained that the catheter would not need to be inserted repeatedly.

Is this the right stage of illness to make the decision?

It is important to consider problems at the appropriate stage of a disease. For example there is usually a stage when a wheelchair becomes extremely useful for a patient with motor neurone disease. But if a wheelchair is discussed too early it can be demoralising or frightening, and if it is left too late it can cause unnecessary suffering and handicap. For cancer patients decision-points often come at times of deterioration, whereas making big decisions may be inappropriate when their condition is stable.

Has the importance of an underlying assumption changed?

A man of 55 with advanced cancer of the lung was on warfarin for valvular heart disease. In the last fortnight of his life he developed ischaemic gangrene of both feet which was very painful. The pain responded only partly to opioids, and he had 4 days and nights of uncontrolled pain. It had been decided from the beginning of his illness that NSAIDs could not be used because he was on warfarin and he also had a recent history of peptic ulceration – a sensible decision, because NSAIDs would have risked gastrointestinal haemorrhage. But priorities had now changed. Warfarin to prevent thrombo-embolic problems in the future was no longer important compared to the pain from his gangrenous feet. The warfarin was stopped and a subcutaneous infusion of diclofenac 150mg per day was started, and his pain virtually disappeared.

Is this the right time?

It is tempting for professionals to initiate discussions when it suits us, but it may not be the appropriate time. For example a man with advanced cancer of the pancreas had two young sons, aged 7 and 9. He was visited by a Macmillan nurse, who asked his wife what their children understood about the illness. She started to talk about it, then paused and said, "I <u>do</u> want to talk about this, but I have to go and pick the children up from the school playground shortly, and I don't want to start crying just at the moment".

Does a previous decision need challenging?

Decisions or diagnoses that get written in the medical notes tend to remain unchallenged. When facing difficult problems it can be important to re-consider previous decisions.

Who has the power?

A divorced woman of 48 with uncontrolled pain from far-advanced cancer of the cervix developed vomiting and was found to have advanced renal failure due to ureteric obstruction. It was decided by the oncology team that this was a terminal event and she went home to die. A visit from a hospice doctor the following day led to a discussion about her main concerns and priorities, and she talked about the importance of seeing her daughter through her exams. She asked about treatment options and ureteric stents were mentioned. It was explained that prolonging her life led to the probability of worsening pain and the possibility of fistula formation. She decided swiftly that she wanted ureteric stents (if technically possible) and she returned to hospital and stents were inserted later the same day. She lived for several more months.

Does the patient have different attitudes to us?

Patients often have different perspectives to their carers, and it is easy to make incorrect assumptions. For example a hospice study in 1997 (of 23 patients and 18 nurses) showed that terminally ill patients accepted the idea of invasive procedures more readily than their nurses. Another study in 1990 also showed that cancer patients have different attitudes to healthy people. It is dangerous to guess or assume what is right for a patient. Every patient is different.

DIFFERING ATTITUDES

<u>Question</u>: "*What percentage chance* of controlling symptoms would encourage you to undergo chemotherapy which would probably cause side-effects of nausea, vomiting and tiredness?"

	COMMONEST REPLY
100 healthy people said:	50%
303 cancer nurses said:	25%
390 GPs said:	25%
148 cancer doctors said:	25%
100 cancer patients said:	1%

Slevin et al 1990

ATTITUDES TO ILLNESS

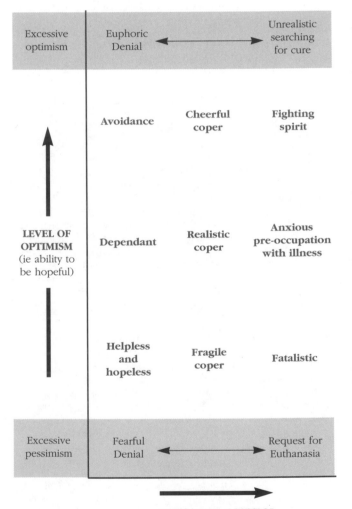

Excessive optimism	Euphoric Denial	⟷	Unrealistic searching for cure
	Avoidance	Cheerful coper	Fighting spirit
LEVEL OF OPTIMISM (ie ability to be hopeful)	Dependant	Realistic coper	Anxious pre-occupation with illness
	Helpless and hopeless	Fragile coper	Fatalistic
Excessive pessimism	Fearful Denial	⟷	Request for Euthanasia

DESIRE FOR CONTROL
(and involvement in medical decision-making)

What attitudes do patient's adopt?

The way patients adjust to serious illness falls into certain patterns. Greer and Watson (1987) identified 5 common adjustment styles: Fighting spirit, avoidance, fatalism, helpless and hopeless and anxious preoccupation. They also produced some evidence that adopting a fighting spirit may prolong survival from cancer. This may be true, and it can be an effective way of coping at certain stages of illness, but it can become unhelpful if taken to extremes. The attitudes they described can be defined in terms of two factors: Level of hopefulness and degree of control wanted (see chart opposite).

What is the best attitude to serious illness?

The best attitude to serious illness is to be half-way between hopeful and hopeless (ie realistic) and half-way between total independence and depending on professionals to do everything (ie willing to participate in the care). This is the central position on the graph opposite (labelled "realistic coper") and this is the position we tend to try and help patients move towards in terms of their attitudes to illness.

Can attitudes be altered?

Attitudes depend partly on personality and it is very difficult to change personality. But attitudes also depend on life experiences and contact with other people. There are usually good reasons underlying a person's attitudes to their illness, often relating to previous life experiences. For example an intelligent woman of 73 hid her breast cancer for 5 years, not because of denial, but because of several bad experiences with the medical care of her parents who both had cancer. She was fatalistic that involvement of doctors would only make her situation worse. However once she had an opportunity to share her feelings in some detail with a doctor she developed some trust and began to share in the medical decision-making with her professional carers (*see* Denial).

Is it possible to increase optimism?

If a patient begins to feel cared for, safe and listened to they often begin to feel less hopeless about the future. Hope is always possible, but needs to be realistic, ideally in the form of realistic short-term goals. (*See* Spiritual distress.)

AUDIT

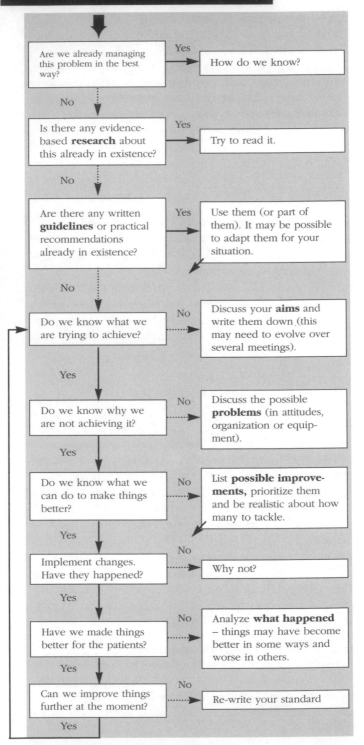

Are we already managing this problem in the best way? — **Yes** → How do we know?

No

Is there any evidence-based **research** about this already in existence? — **Yes** → Try to read it.

No

Are there any written **guidelines** or practical recommendations already in existence? — **Yes** → Use them (or part of them). It may be possible to adapt them for your situation.

No

Do we know what we are trying to achieve? — **No** → Discuss your **aims** and write them down (this may need to evolve over several meetings).

Yes

Do we know why we are not achieving it? — **No** → Discuss the possible **problems** (in attitudes, organization or equipment).

Yes

Do we know what we can do to make things better? — **No** → List **possible improvements,** prioritize them and be realistic about how many to tackle.

Yes

Implement changes. Have they happened? — **No** → Why not?

Yes

Have we made things better for the patients? — **No** → Analyze **what happened** – things may have become better in some ways and worse in others.

Yes

Can we improve things further at the moment? — **No** → Re-write your standard

Yes

What is audit?

Clinical audit is a way of examining our activities to encourage best practice. It provides feedback about what we do and how it compares with our peers, and helps us to change our environment, our systems or ourselves in order to improve patient care.

Clinical audit is not an exercise in data collection. It is simply a way of providing best care in the face of limitations (environment, resources and our own knowledge).

Simply distributing documents does not lead to change, we all need support to change bad habits.

What is the difference between audit and research?

Research leads to evidence which leads to guidelines which lead to audit. On the other hand audit may uncover areas of ignorance of interest to researchers.

DIFFERENCES BETWEEN RESEARCH AND AUDIT	
RESEARCH	**AUDIT**
• One-off project	• On-going activity
• Collects complex data	• Uses routine data
• Discovers the right treatment	• Ensures the right treatment happens
• Uses large (statistically significant) samples	• Uses small samples
• Generalisations <u>can</u> be made from a particular research project	• Generalisations <u>cannot</u> be made from a particular audit project

Are guidelines available?

Guidelines shape the research available into a body of recommendations that reflect the realities of everyday clinical practice. Producing authoritative guidelines is difficult (and ensuring they are followed is even more difficult). Don't re-invent the wheel, base your guidelines on those developed elsewhere. (*See* Guidelines.)

How do we start?

A written standard should be developed (using guidelines, if available) setting out agreed policies (eg "patients should have pain controlled within one week") and practice should be reviewed from time to time to see whether the standard is being achieved. A designated member of the team should be responsible for ensuring that monitoring occurs.

What is the audit cycle?

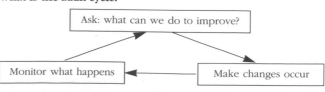

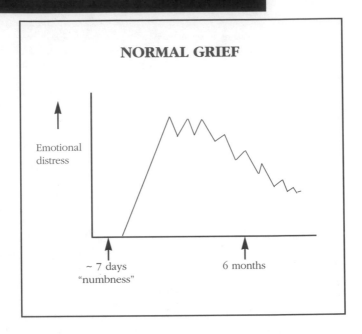

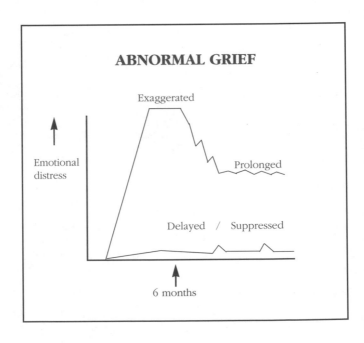

Should bereavement counselling be offered?

Bereavement is a universal experience, but 30% of people develop significant depression for a time afterwards. Resources do not usually allow an offer of support to everyone. Those at risk of abnormal grief reactions should be normally followed up (especially the confused elderly, those with learning disabilities and children) plus any others who seem at risk.

INCREASED RISK OF ABNORMAL GRIEF

- Children
- Learning disabilities
- Confused elderly – Elderly male widower
- Very dependent
- Ambivalent relationship
- Multiple prior bereavements
- Previous depression
- Low self esteem
- Poor social support
- Other life crises
- Inability to carry out valued religious rituals at time of death
- Sudden and unexpected death
- Death of young person
- Stigmatised deaths – Such as AIDS, suicide
- Culpable deaths

Is the grief abnormal?

Grief can be abnormal in different ways (exaggerated, prolonged, delayed). Abnormal grief is a matter of judgement, and partly cultural (eg a West Indian lying in the corridor wailing may be more "normal" than a stockbroker from Esher doing the same thing).

If the bereaved person develops significant psychological problems refer for formal bereavement therapy from a trained professional (counsellor, social worker, psychologist, psychiatrist).

BEREAVEMENT THERAPY

- Time and space to grieve
- Explanation of normal emotions
- Expression of negative emotions
- Discussion of changing needs
- Exploring previous losses
- Skilful ending of therapy (another loss)
- Re-referral at difficult periods

BLEEDING

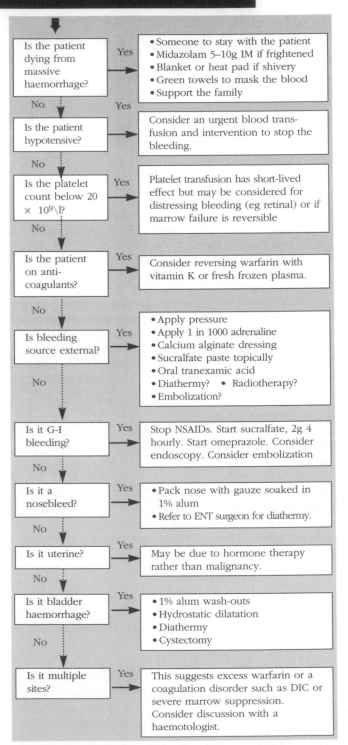

Is the patient dying from massive haemorrhage? — Yes →
- Someone to stay with the patient
- Midazolam 5–10g IM if frightened
- Blanket or heat pad if shivery
- Green towels to mask the blood
- Support the family

No ↓

Is the patient hypotensive? — Yes →
Consider an urgent blood transfusion and intervention to stop the bleeding.

No ↓

Is the platelet count below 20 × 10^9\l? — Yes →
Platelet transfusion has short-lived effect but may be considered for distressing bleeding (eg retinal) or if marrow failure is reversible

No ↓

Is the patient on anti-coagulants? — Yes →
Consider reversing warfarin with vitamin K or fresh frozen plasma.

No ↓

Is bleeding source external? — Yes →
- Apply pressure
- Apply 1 in 1000 adrenaline
- Calcium alginate dressing
- Sucralfate paste topically
- Oral tranexamic acid
- Diathermy? • Radiotherapy?
- Embolization?

No ↓

Is it G-I bleeding? — Yes →
Stop NSAIDs. Start sucralfate, 2g 4 hourly. Start omeprazole. Consider endoscopy. Consider embolization

No ↓

Is it a nosebleed? — Yes →
- Pack nose with gauze soaked in 1% alum
- Refer to ENT surgeon for diathermy.

No ↓

Is it uterine? — Yes →
May be due to hormone therapy rather than malignancy.

No ↓

Is it bladder haemorrhage? — Yes →
- 1% alum wash-outs
- Hydrostatic dilatation
- Diathermy
- Cystectomy

No ↓

Is it multiple sites? — Yes →
This suggests excess warfarin or a coagulation disorder such as DIC or severe marrow suppression. Consider discussion with a haemotologist.

Can the bleeding be controlled?

There are a number of ways of controlling bleeding (that are often overlooked). Tranexamic acid can be very effective, other methods are described in the flow chart opposite.

Is the patient frightened?

Even very minor bleeding terrifies some patients who see it as life threatening. A bit of explanation can be very therapeutic.

Is oral iron indicated?

Long-term low-grade bleeding such as haematuria depletes iron stores and the patient should be on oral iron supplements.

Is a blood transfusion indicated?

Blood transfusion is only indicated if the bleeding has been controlled, otherwise it simply worsens the haemorrhage.

Is radiotherapy indicated?

Radiotherapy can effectively control haemorrhage and should always be considered in tumours of the lung, bladder, uterus, vagina or rectum.

Is platelet transfusion indicated?

Marrow involvement that has reduced the platelet count to below $10 \times 10^9 \backslash l$ causes spontaneous haemorrhages (purpura or bruising may be visible). Platelet transfusion is only effective in controlling bleeding for 2 or 3 days but may be indicated even in the terminal phase if the effects of bleeding is particularly devastating (eg retinal haemorrhages).

Is heavy terminal bleeding likely?

A patient who has invasion of a major artery such as carotid or femoral and has had some warning bleeds may die from massive haemorrhage. Have green towels available (which reduce the impact of red blood on white sheets) and if it happens someone should stay with the patient. Somebody else should draw up diamorphine and midazolam but should ask the patient before giving it. If masive haemorrhage is a very strong possibility the timing of explanation and fore-warning to both the patient and family is a matter of judgement.

BOREDOM

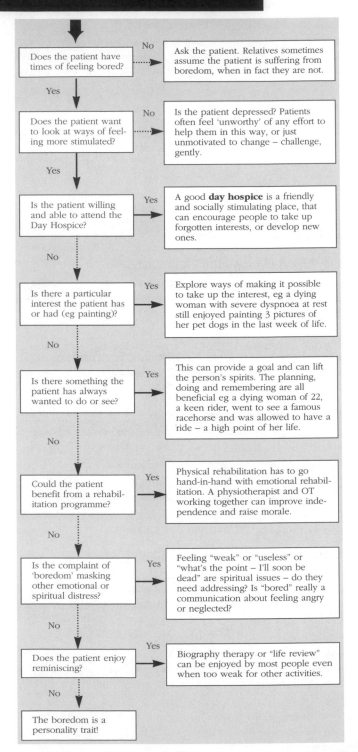

Does the patient have times of feeling bored? — **No** → Ask the patient. Relatives sometimes assume the patient is suffering from boredom, when in fact they are not.

Yes ↓

Does the patient want to look at ways of feeling more stimulated? — **No** → Is the patient depressed? Patients often feel 'unworthy' of any effort to help them in this way, or just unmotivated to change – challenge, gently.

Yes ↓

Is the patient willing and able to attend the Day Hospice? — **Yes** → A good **day hospice** is a friendly and socially stimulating place, that can encourage people to take up forgotten interests, or develop new ones.

No ↓

Is there a particular interest the patient has or had (eg painting)? — **Yes** → Explore ways of making it possible to take up the interest, eg a dying woman with severe dyspnoea at rest still enjoyed painting 3 pictures of her pet dogs in the last week of life.

No ↓

Is there something the patient has always wanted to do or see? — **Yes** → This can provide a goal and can lift the person's spirits. The planning, doing and remembering are all beneficial eg a dying woman of 22, a keen rider, went to see a famous racehorse and was allowed to have a ride – a high point of her life.

No ↓

Could the patient benefit from a rehabilitation programme? — **Yes** → Physical rehabilitation has to go hand-in-hand with emotional rehabilitation. A physiotherapist and OT working together can improve independence and raise morale.

No ↓

Is the complaint of 'boredom' masking other emotional or spiritual distress? — **Yes** → Feeling "weak" or "useless" or "what's the point – I'll soon be dead" are spiritual issues – do they need addressing? Is "bored" really a communication about feeling angry or neglected?

No ↓

Does the patient enjoy reminiscing? — **Yes** → Biography therapy or "life review" can be enjoyed by most people even when too weak for other activities.

No ↓

The boredom is a personality trait!

50

Would physiotherapy help?

Sometimes patients have lost confidence and independence because family members have been too kind. A graded approach to rehabilitation can build up a patients self confidence and achieving short term goals often boasts morale and prevents boredom. Opportunities for rehabilitation can be lost if professionals lack imagination or initiative depriving some patients of what one carer called "those precious moments of triumph".

Would occupational therapy help?

Occupational therapy can be defined as science of healing by occupation. Loss of independence and role can result in social death prior to biological death. Occupation therapy can help a patient become purposefully engaged again in regular and familiar life experiences which restores the patient's self-esteem and helps them to adapt to new activities and roles. Occupational therapy enables social rehabilitation. It can also help the patient to take up therapeutic activities such as arts, crafts, poetry or music, ideally short term projects that are easy to pick up and set down and have pleasing results.

Would the patient benefit from the Day Hospice?

Day Hospice brings opportunities for socialising and group activities and games as well as providing an informal atmosphere where patients can support each other.

Would reminiscence therapy help?

Reminiscence is a natural and enjoyable past time which can be especially helpful when weakness prevents any other activities. Encouraging reminiscence helps the patient to feel known as themselves and a sense of meaning can be derived from memories of past loves and past achievements. It integrates their present experiences into the context of their whole life. Formal interviewing and tape recording the patient's life story enables it to be transcribed and produced as a written archive (to be left by the patient) which patient's and relatives can find very enjoyable.

BREAKING BAD NEWS

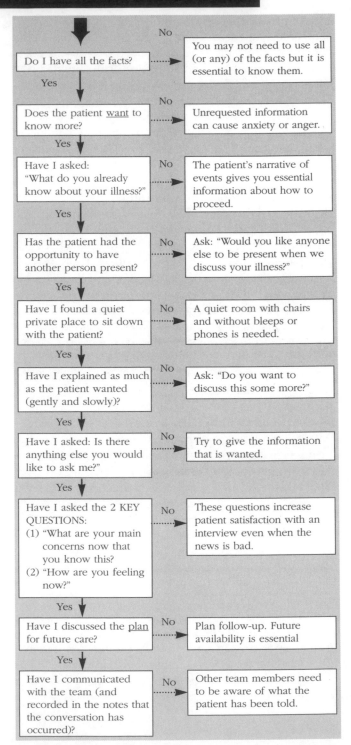

Do I have all the facts? — No → You may not need to use all (or any) of the facts but it is essential to know them.

Yes ↓

Does the patient want to know more? — No → Unrequested information can cause anxiety or anger.

Yes ↓

Have I asked: "What do you already know about your illness?" — No → The patient's narrative of events gives you essential information about how to proceed.

Yes ↓

Has the patient had the opportunity to have another person present? — No → Ask: "Would you like anyone else to be present when we discuss your illness?"

Yes ↓

Have I found a quiet private place to sit down with the patient? — No → A quiet room with chairs and without bleeps or phones is needed.

Yes ↓

Have I explained as much as the patient wanted (gently and slowly)? — No → Ask: "Do you want to discuss this some more?"

Yes ↓

Have I asked: Is there anything else you would like to ask me?" — No → Try to give the information that is wanted.

Yes ↓

Have I asked the 2 KEY QUESTIONS:
(1) "What are your main concerns now that you know this?
(2) "How are you feeling now?" — No → These questions increase patient satisfaction with an interview even when the news is bad.

Yes ↓

Have I discussed the plan for future care? — No → Plan follow-up. Future availability is essential

Yes ↓

Have I communicated with the team (and recorded in the notes that the conversation has occurred)? — No → Other team members need to be aware of what the patient has been told.

Is bad news likely?

If bad news is expected it can be very helpful to prepare yourself and the patient (eg before a laparotomy for suspected cancer) by having a dialogue about what sort of information they would find helpful, how much they would want to know and whether they would want anybody else with them when the situation was discussed.

Do I know the facts?

Before explaining bad news it is very important that you understand the facts clearly, even though you may not need to discuss them. This gives you confidence that you are clear about the situation and enables you to focus more on the way you are saying and conveying information rather than information itself.

Have I asked questions?

Breaking bad news should start by asking questions to find out how much the patient already knows and wants to know. Getting a feel for the patient's attitudes.

Is this the right moment?

It may be better to defer the meeting to a more appropriate time e.g. if the patient has got symptoms such as pain or nausea or if it would be appropriate to have another person there such as the patient's partner (e.g. "I would be very happy to discuss this with you in detail but I think we should make another appointment when I can give you more time").

Have I given the right amount of information?

The right amount of information lies somewhere between too little and too much and it is a matter of judgement. Too little leaves the patient confused and dissatisfied and too much leaves the patient anxious. Keep checking with the patient whether the amount of information you have given is adequate.

Have I conveyed empathy?

Conveying empathy is the key to a satisfactory interview. Having explained the situation check out with the patient how it has changed their perspective and their feelings (e.g. How do you feel about what I have just explained ? Does it feel a shock?).

Should I see the patient again?

Follow-up is important. Most patient cannot take in very much information when they are emotionally shocked or distressed and need time to piece together the complex jig-saw of their altered future, and need opportunities to talk it over with professionals (on more than one occasion.)

CARERS

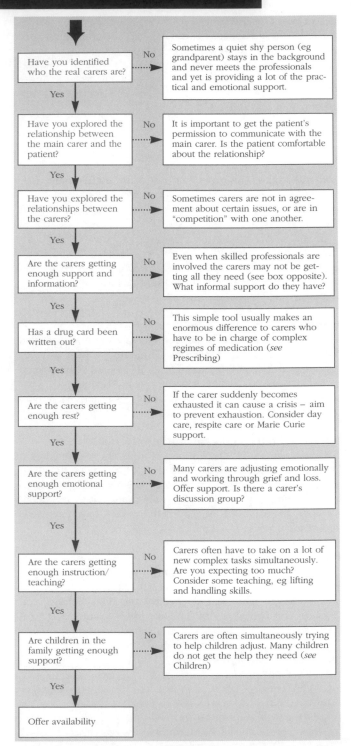

Have you identified who the real carers are? — No → Sometimes a quiet shy person (eg grandparent) stays in the background and never meets the professionals and yet is providing a lot of the practical and emotional support.

↓ Yes

Have you explored the relationship between the main carer and the patient? — No → It is important to get the patient's permission to communicate with the main carer. Is the patient comfortable about the relationship?

↓ Yes

Have you explored the relationships between the carers? — No → Sometimes carers are not in agreement about certain issues, or are in "competition" with one another.

↓ Yes

Are the carers getting enough support and information? — No → Even when skilled professionals are involved the carers may not be getting all they need (see box opposite). What informal support do they have?

↓ Yes

Has a drug card been written out? — No → This simple tool usually makes an enormous difference to carers who have to be in charge of complex regimes of medication (*see* Prescribing)

↓ Yes

Are the carers getting enough rest? — No → If the carer suddenly becomes exhausted it can cause a crisis – aim to prevent exhaustion. Consider day care, respite care or Marie Curie support.

↓ Yes

Are the carers getting enough emotional support? — No → Many carers are adjusting emotionally and working through grief and loss. Offer support. Is there a carer's discussion group?

↓ Yes

Are the carers getting enough instruction/teaching? — No → Carers often have to take on a lot of new complex tasks simultaneously. Are you expecting too much? Consider some teaching, eg lifting and handling skills.

↓ Yes

Are children in the family getting enough support? — No → Carers are often simultaneously trying to help children adjust. Many children do not get the help they need (*see* Children)

↓ Yes

Offer availability

DECISION-MAKING FOR CARERS

"On many occasions my wife was discharged with maybe a dozen drugs all designed in some way to help her with the treatment surrounding her terminal cancer and no doubt most of which could cause serious harm if administered unwisely.

Many drugs may be prescribed with little explanation other than dosage and the information sheet. Information sheets often come with drugs collected from high street chemists but not usually when sourced at hospital pharmacies.

You may say all I had to do was ask and yes I could ring up our GP or Consultant, and did do so occasionally, usually at times when my wife was in severe pain. However I was aware of the importance of the scarce resources and it is just not possible to speak to the relevant medical professionals every time a decision is needed.

At the end of the day rightly or wrongly it falls to the carer to make a decision concerning what medication to issue especially on those all too frequent occasions when it isn't possible to follow exactly the doctor's instructions. How is the carer to know where to draw the line between missing a dose and not following the course of medication?.

I wanted to get it right, to give my wife the best chance of a better quality of life. Maybe the very fact that I exhibited more than the average commitment to looking after my wife led to the perception that I was capable of making any necessary decisions, a victim of my own success.

Towards the end of my wife's life we did get more help from District Nurses but all too often they were not able to answer my concerns although, of course, they undertook to find out on my behalf.

Surely I cannot be the only person to feel such pressure. After all, what is good for the carer has got to be good for the patient."

Graham Watson
– a carer

CHEMOTHERAPY

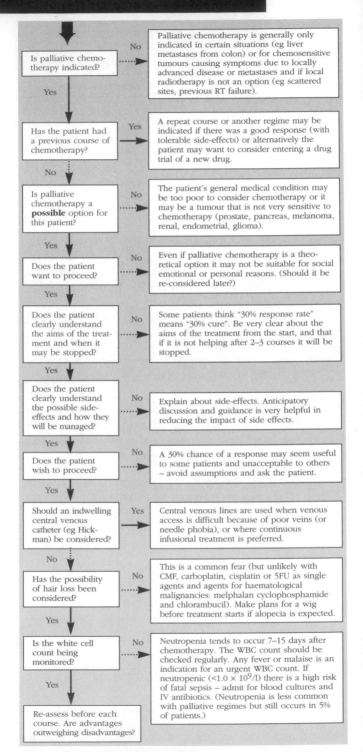

Is palliative chemotherapy indicated? — No → Palliative chemotherapy is generally only indicated in certain situations (eg liver metastases from colon) or for chemosensitive tumours causing symptoms due to locally advanced disease or metastases and if local radiotherapy is not an option (eg scattered sites, previous RT failure).

↓ Yes

Has the patient had a previous course of chemotherapy? — Yes → A repeat course or another regime may be indicated if there was a good response (with tolerable side-effects) or alternatively the patient may want to consider entering a drug trial of a new drug.

↓ No

Is palliative chemotherapy a possible option for this patient? — No → The patient's general medical condition may be too poor to consider chemotherapy or it may be a tumour that is not very sensitive to chemotherapy (prostate, pancreas, melanoma, renal, endometrial, glioma).

↓ Yes

Does the patient want to proceed? — No → Even if palliative chemotherapy is a theoretical option it may not be suitable for social emotional or personal reasons. (Should it be re-considered later?)

↓ Yes

Does the patient clearly understand the aims of the treatment and when it may be stopped? — No → Some patients think "30% response rate" means "30% cure". Be very clear about the aims of the treatment from the start, and that if it is not helping after 2–3 courses it will be stopped.

↓ Yes

Does the patient clearly understand the possible side-effects and how they will be managed? — No → Explain about side-effects. Anticipatory discussion and guidance is very helpful in reducing the impact of side effects.

↓ Yes

Does the patient wish to proceed? — No → A 30% chance of a response may seem useful to some patients and unacceptable to others – avoid assumptions and ask the patient.

↓ Yes

Should an indwelling central venous catheter (eg Hickman) be considered? — Yes → Central venous lines are used when venous access is difficult because of poor veins (or needle phobia), or where continuous infusional treatment is preferred.

↓ No

Has the possibility of hair loss been considered? — No → This is a common fear (but unlikely with CMF, carboplatin, cisplatin or 5FU as single agents and agents for haematological malignancies: melphalan cyclophosphamide and chlorambucil). Make plans for a wig before treatment starts if alopecia is expected.

↓ Yes

Is the white cell count being monitored? — No → Neutropenia tends to occur 7–15 days after chemotherapy. The WBC count should be checked regularly. Any fever or malaise is an indication for an urgent WBC count. If neutropenic ($<1.0 \times 10^9$/l) there is a high risk of fatal sepsis – admit for blood cultures and IV antibiotics. (Neutropenia is less common with palliative regimes but still occurs in 5% of patients.)

↓ Yes

Re-assess before each course. Are advantages outweighing disadvantages?

Does the patient understand what you mean by the word "chemotherapy"?

Patients are often fearful that "chemotherapy" automatically means intensive regimes of IV chemotherapy a high incidence of severe side- effects such as hair loss, nausea and vomiting and prolonged malaise (and possibly even bone marrow transplant). In fact there are a number of drug regimes which have limited toxicity and are very useful in the palliative care setting including oral melphalan in myeloma, CMF (Cyclophosphamide, Methotrexate and Fluorouracil) in breast cancer, oral etoposide in small cell lung cancer and hormonal therapies.

Is a Hickman line (or other central venous line) needed?

Central venous catheters can be inserted under radiographic control with local anaesthetic. They provide a permanent means of both blood sampling and venous access. The line needs to be flushed weekly with heparinized saline to maintain patentcy. Oral Warfarin 1 mg daily is given to reduce the rate of thrombotic complications. They should be carefully inspected regularly for any signs of infection in patients with neutropenia and if they become infected must be removed. Whenever the line is open the plastic clamps on the line must always be closed to prevent air entering the vein (or, if the patient is supine, blood pouring out) once connected to the syringe or infusion system the clamps are opened. If the line needs to be removed this can be done simply: The clamps should be closed. The Velcro fibrous cuff holding the line in place is dissected free under local anaesthetic, to gently free it from the subcutaneous tissues, after which the tube can easily be pulled out. Pressure should be applied for a few seconds to the site of venous entry in the root of the neck after the catheter is removed.

When should palliative chemotherapy be stopped?

The aim of a course of palliative chemotherapy is to leave the patient feeling better (physically or psychologically) and to cause the tumour to regress. A course of Chemotherapy is normally planned for 2–6 courses (usually 3 weekly) and then reviewed. If the tumour is progressing despite chemotherapy (for example if the serum tumour markers are rising) then chemotherapy should be stopped. It is easier to stop if the aims of treatment were clearly explained from the start.

Tumour Markers

			Normally less than:
HCG	–	Germ cell	4
PSA	–	Prostate	3
AFP	–	Hepatoma, Germ cell	7
CA125	–	Ovary, Breast, Hepatoma	23
CA15-3	–	Breast	28
CA19-9	–	Pancreas, Colon	33
CEA	–	Colon, Breast	4

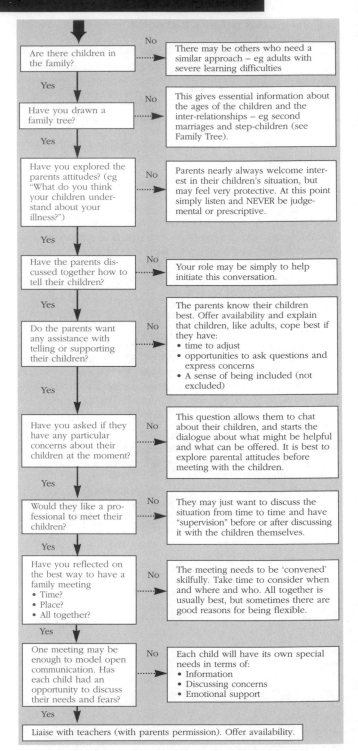

	No	
Are there children in the family?	·····▶	There may be others who need a similar approach – eg adults with severe learning difficulties

Yes

	No	
Have you drawn a family tree?	·····▶	This gives essential information about the ages of the children and the inter-relationships – eg second marriages and step-children (see Family Tree).

Yes

	No	
Have you explored the parents attitudes? (eg "What do you think your children understand about your illness?")	·····▶	Parents nearly always welcome interest in their children's situation, but may feel very protective. At this point simply listen and NEVER be judgemental or prescriptive.

Yes

	No	
Have the parents discussed together how to tell their children?	·····▶	Your role may be simply to help initiate this conversation.

Yes

	No	
Do the parents want any assistance with telling or supporting their children?	·····▶	The parents know their children best. Offer availability and explain that children, like adults, cope best if they have: • time to adjust • opportunities to ask questions and express concerns • A sense of being included (not excluded)

Yes

	No	
Have you asked if they have any particular concerns about their children at the moment?	·····▶	This question allows them to chat about their children, and starts the dialogue about what might be helpful and what can be offered. It is best to explore parental attitudes before meeting with the children.

Yes

	No	
Would they like a professional to meet their children?	·····▶	They may just want to discuss the situation from time to time and have "supervision" before or after discussing it with the children themselves.

Yes

	No	
Have you reflected on the best way to have a family meeting • Time? • Place? • All together?	·····▶	The meeting needs to be 'convened' skilfully. Take time to consider when and where and who. All together is usually best, but sometimes there are good reasons for being flexible.

Yes

	No	
One meeting may be enough to model open communication. Has each child had an opportunity to discuss their needs and fears?	·····▶	Each child will have its own special needs in terms of: • Information • Discussing concerns • Emotional support

Yes

Liaise with teachers (with parents permission). Offer availability.

How old are the children?
Children's needs depend on age. The 3 main age-groups have slightly different needs: Under 5, 5-12, and teenagers (although individual children vary). Information and language needs to be tailored to children's developmental age and experience of death.

Are the children getting enough information?
Parents underestimate the impact of illness on their children, and often report little evidence of emotional distress in their children. Children themselves however report being ignored and experiencing a lot of emotional symptoms. Many parents do not discuss the fears and uncertainties of illness or death with their children, in the hope that this is protective. But the children then feel isolated, confused and frightened (and later on resentful that they did not know).

How can professionals help?
Families facing life-threatening illness commonly have difficulty talking about it. Children's problems often get minimised by overwhelmed parents. Parents often need considerable support when dealing with their children's feelings. Doctors need to discuss with parents at an early stage how and what children should be told. Once adults realise that open discussion of fears and uncertainties leaves them feeling better, it is easier for them to see it might also help their children. Explain the principle of helping children (clear, truthful explanation and open discussion). Negotiate with the parents how much professional help (if any) they want for their children.

How do you talk with children?
Children need clear (repeated) explanations of the simple truth. Using euphemisms (eg "he's gone on a journey" or "he's gone to sleep") can cause problems later (when people want to go on a real journey or go to sleep) and are confusing. Young children communicate through play.

What do children need to reduce their anxieties?
Children need knowledge of the illness, information from their parents, a feeling of inclusion and involvement, clear explanations, to be able to help, opportunities to ask questions, permission to say how they really feel, awareness of sadness in others, guidance about what to do and prompt explanation if changes occur.

How much explanation is needed?
More than you think. Just stating what seems obvious (to you) can be extremely helpful to children eg at the right time explaining what death looks like can be very re-assuring ("The skin changes colour, sometimes a bit blue and then white, the breathing sometimes gets noisy, the heart slows down and eventually stops, brain waves stop, then the person does not move any more.")

Should books be offered?
There are many useful books (and games) to help children adjust to grief. Give the book to a parent first "to see if the child might find it helpful" because it is essential for the parent(s) to be comfortable with it. Be careful not to offer a book as a substitute for emotional support and counselling.

COGNITIVE THERAPY

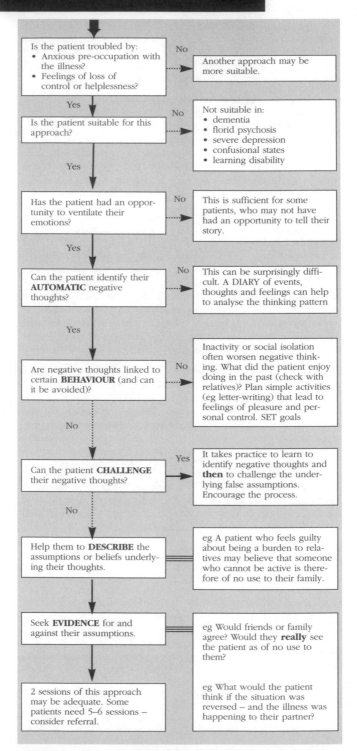

Is the patient troubled by:
- Anxious pre-occupation with the illness?
- Feelings of loss of control or helplessness?

No → Another approach may be more suitable.

Yes ↓

Is the patient suitable for this approach?

No → Not suitable in:
- dementia
- florid psychosis
- severe depression
- confusional states
- learning disability

Yes ↓

Has the patient had an opportunity to ventilate their emotions?

No → This is sufficient for some patients, who may not have had an opportunity to tell their story.

Yes ↓

Can the patient identify their **AUTOMATIC** negative thoughts?

No → This can be surprisingly difficult. A DIARY of events, thoughts and feelings can help to analyse the thinking pattern

Yes ↓

Are negative thoughts linked to certain **BEHAVIOUR** (and can it be avoided)?

No → Inactivity or social isolation often worsen negative thinking. What did the patient enjoy doing in the past (check with relatives)? Plan simple activities (eg letter-writing) that lead to feelings of pleasure and personal control. SET goals

No ↓

Can the patient **CHALLENGE** their negative thoughts?

Yes → It takes practice to learn to identify negative thoughts and **then** to challenge the underlying false assumptions. Encourage the process.

No ↓

Help them to **DESCRIBE** the assumptions or beliefs underlying their thoughts.

eg A patient who feels guilty about being a burden to relatives may believe that someone who cannot be active is therefore of no use to their family.

↓

Seek **EVIDENCE** for and against their assumptions.

eg Would friends or family agree? Would they **really** see the patient as of no use to them?

↓

2 sessions of this approach may be adequate. Some patients need 5–6 sessions – consider referral.

eg What would the patient think if the situation was reversed – and the illness was happening to their partner?

COGNITIVE THERAPY

What is cognitive therapy?
We all make internal (unspoken) assumptions about what is happening around us and to us. If our automatic thoughts are based on incorrect assumptions or fantasies they can cause anxiety or depression or both. When this unrealistic thinking is the main problem then cognitive therapy can be very effective in helping a patient gradually feel more in control of their thinking.

> "**Psychological problems** are not necessarily the product of mysterious, impenetrable forces but may result from commonplace processes such as faulty learning, making incorrect inferences on the basis of inadequate or incorrect information and not distinguishing adequately between imagination and reality"
>
> *Aaron Beck, 1976*

Is the patient suitable for this approach?
The patient needs to be verbally competent and willing to verbalise their distress. It seems most useful when the main problems relate to feelings of loss of control or anxious preoccupation with the illness or low self esteem (eg "I am useless" "I am a burden", "I'd be better off dead").

Can the patient identify their negative thoughts?
Negative thinking is based on incorrect assumptions (e.g. "ill people are worthless"). Teach the patient to identify then challenge (reality-test) their assumptions. What evidence do they have for their beliefs?

Is the patient participating in decisions about their care?
Learning about the treatment, and being involved in decision-making can lead to a willingness to carry on life or as normally as possible, and an optimism that can reduce habitual negative thoughts.

What activities result in feeling good and in control?
There may be activities that the patient used to enjoy but has now abandoned, or a history of activities that contradict their present negative view of themselves. New simple activities can reverse the feeling "I can't do what I did so I may as well do nothing". Positive activities often lead to more positive thinking.

See also: Counselling, Crisis Intervention, Support

61

CONFUSION

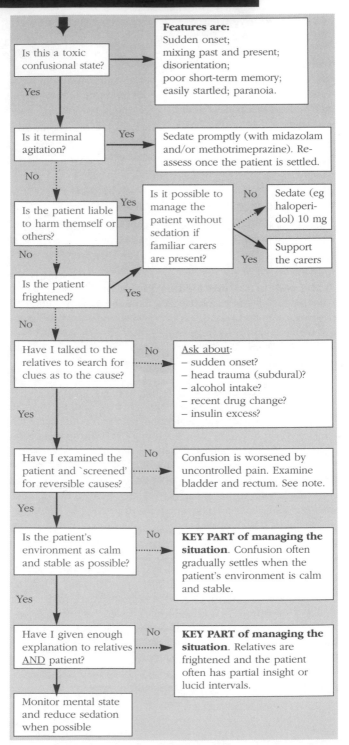

Is this a toxic confusional state?

Features are:
Sudden onset;
mixing past and present;
disorientation;
poor short-term memory;
easily startled; paranoia.

Yes

Is it terminal agitation? — Yes → Sedate promptly (with midazolam and/or methotrimeprazine). Re-assess once the patient is settled.

No

Is the patient liable to harm themselves or others? — Yes → Is it possible to manage the patient without sedation if familiar carers are present? — No → Sedate (eg haloperidol) 10 mg

— Yes → Support the carers

No

Is the patient frightened? — Yes →

No

Have I talked to the relatives to search for clues as to the cause? — No → Ask about:
– sudden onset?
– head trauma (subdural)?
– alcohol intake?
– recent drug change?
– insulin excess?

Yes

Have I examined the patient and `screened' for reversible causes? — No → Confusion is worsened by uncontrolled pain. Examine bladder and rectum. See note.

Yes

Is the patient's environment as calm and stable as possible? — No → **KEY PART of managing the situation**. Confusion often gradually settles when the patient's environment is calm and stable.

Yes

Have I given enough explanation to relatives __AND__ patient? — No → **KEY PART of managing the situation**. Relatives are frightened and the patient often has partial insight or lucid intervals.

Monitor mental state and reduce sedation when possible

Is it confusion or dementia?

Confusion can be reversible but dementia is not. Confusion is usually of sudden onset, over days and dementia is of gradual onset, over months. Confusion is usually obvious (rambling speech, poor memory for recent events, disorientation, drowsy yet easily startled) but remember that the patient may have both dementia and confusion, or neither – they may just be deaf, grumpy and out of their normal environment.

Is it terminal agitation?

If the patient is dying, confused and agitated (physical and mentally) it is usually best (for both the patient and the relatives) to sedate promptly (with midazolam and\or methotrimeprazine), then re-assess the situation and consider reducing sedation. High doses may be needed. Is there a reversible reason (eg urinary retention).

Is it alcohol withdrawal?

Sudden severe agitation suggests 'delirium tremens' due to alcohol withdrawal in an alcoholic. The best solution in advanced illness is often to restore a reasonable alcohol intake.

Is there a reversible cause?

Ask relatives about recent drug changes, examine carefully (especially bladder and rectum) and check blood glucose, calcium, urea electrolytes. Send a MSU to exclude UTI.

Is a CT scan indicated?

Consider a CT scan if there has been a head injury within recent weeks, (a subdural haematoma may be treatable) or if there are neurological signs suggestive of brain metastases

Is the patient lucid at times?

Lucid intervals often occur (usually in the morning) when it is possible to converse with the patient, and discover their wishes about management options.

Is the environment calm?

The most important part of management is to create a calm stable environment (quiet, dim lighting, familiar faces). A familiar relative to sit with the patient can be very calming (but the relative may need a lot of support). The patient may need admitting from home. Confusion is the most difficult symptom to manage at home, because it tends to erode the carer's emotional energy for coping – consider admission.

Is sedation needed?

Confusion may not be distressing (and we then tend to say the patient is "pleasantly confused") but it may be very frightening. Acknowledging the patient's fear can help to calm the patient.

Are the relatives getting enough support?

Confusion is frightening for the relatives. Explanation helps (likely cause, likely course of events etc).

CONSENT

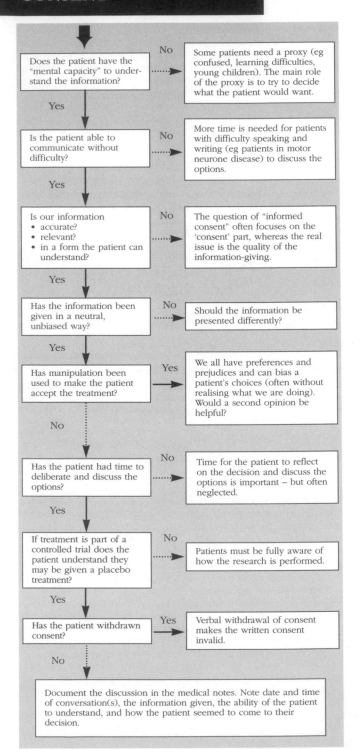

Does the patient have the "mental capacity" to understand the information? → **No** → Some patients need a proxy (eg confused, learning difficulties, young children). The main role of the proxy is to try to decide what the patient would want.

Yes ↓

Is the patient able to communicate without difficulty? → **No** → More time is needed for patients with difficulty speaking and writing (eg patients in motor neurone disease) to discuss the options.

Yes ↓

Is our information
• accurate?
• relevant?
• in a form the patient can understand? → **No** → The question of "informed consent" often focuses on the 'consent' part, whereas the real issue is the quality of the information-giving.

Yes ↓

Has the information been given in a neutral, unbiased way? → **No** → Should the information be presented differently?

Yes ↓

Has manipulation been used to make the patient accept the treatment? → **Yes** → We all have preferences and prejudices and can bias a patient's choices (often without realising what we are doing). Would a second opinion be helpful?

No ↓

Has the patient had time to deliberate and discuss the options? → **No** → Time for the patient to reflect on the decision and discuss the options is important – but often neglected.

Yes ↓

If treatment is part of a controlled trial does the patient understand they may be given a placebo treatment? → **No** → Patients must be fully aware of how the research is performed.

Yes ↓

Has the patient withdrawn consent? → **Yes** → Verbal withdrawal of consent makes the written consent invalid.

No ↓

Document the discussion in the medical notes. Note date and time of conversation(s), the information given, the ability of the patient to understand, and how the patient seemed to come to their decision.

Is the patient competent to make a decision about their treatment?

There is no simple test to detect whether a patient has the mental capacity to understand. The main point is to decide whether the patient can retain information long enough to make a decision. The best way to decide this is to get them to repeat the information you give them. It is sometimes helpful to involve next of kin either to help in decision-making or to witness the decision.

What information is needed?

Patients should be offered information about:
- benefits
- risks
- alternative options
- results of non-treatment

There is a difference between being given information and understanding information. Patients also have some responsibilities to ask for the information they want.

How much information should be given?

For most treatments (eg prescribing a drug) we give information, and the patient's consent is usually implied and assumed. The amount of information we give (and whether we ask for written consent) relates to the level of risk involved in the treatment .

Should every possible risk be explained?

Inadequate information can be distressing, but over detailed information can also be distressing. U.S. doctors now sometimes give patients information in writing about every possible risk of a treatment (for legal reasons). There is no correct answer to the question of how much detail to give - it is a matter of judgement, and needs to be appropriate to the patient's level of intelligence, their situation and the degree of risk.

Does consent for clinical research differ?

The same principles apply, but because of the risk of subtle pressures on the patient to take part in a trial, it must be made clear that they are free to withdraw without explanation or obstacle at any stage (especially if it is a placebo controlled trial) and that this will not prejudice their future care, and also it is especially important to involve the next-of-kin in the decision (with, not instead of, the patient).

See also: Assumptions

CONSTIPATION

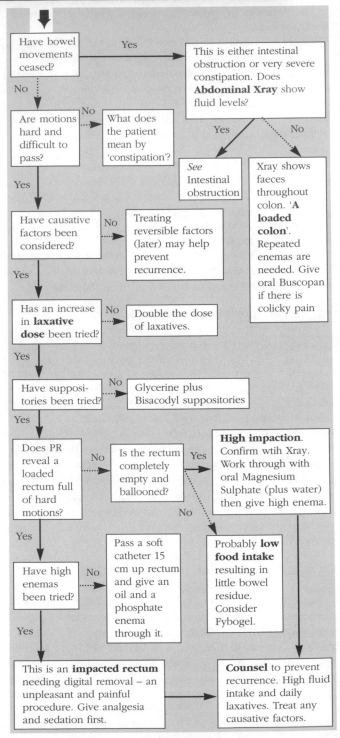

Have bowel movements ceased?
— Yes → This is either intestinal obstruction or very severe constipation. Does **Abdominal Xray** show fluid levels?

No ↓

Are motions hard and difficult to pass?
— No ┄→ What does the patient mean by 'constipation'?

From "Abdominal Xray":
- Yes → *See* Intestinal obstruction
- No ┄→ Xray shows faeces throughout colon. '**A loaded colon**'. Repeated enemas are needed. Give oral Buscopan if there is colicky pain

Yes ↓

Have causative factors been considered?
— No ┄→ Treating reversible factors (later) may help prevent recurrence.

Yes ↓

Has an increase in **laxative dose** been tried?
— No ┄→ Double the dose of laxatives.

Yes ↓

Have suppositories been tried?
— No ┄→ Glycerine plus Bisacodyl suppositories

Yes ↓

Does PR reveal a loaded rectum full of hard motions?
— No ┄→ Is the rectum completely empty and ballooned?
  - Yes → **High impaction**. Confirm wtih Xray. Work through with oral Magnesium Sulphate (plus water) then give high enema.
  - No ┄→ Probably **low food intake** resulting in little bowel residue. Consider Fybogel.

Yes ↓

Have high enemas been tried?
— No ┄→ Pass a soft catheter 15 cm up rectum and give an oil and a phosphate enema through it.

Yes ↓

This is an **impacted rectum** needing digital removal – an unpleasant and painful procedure. Give analgesia and sedation first.
→ **Counsel** to prevent recurrence. High fluid intake and daily laxatives. Treat any causative factors.

CONSTIPATION

Is the patient constipated?
Some patients use "constipation" to mean less frequent bowel movement, but constipation means difficulty passing motions – usually because they are hard. It is a common problem and can be extremely distressing. One patient wrote in her diary – "Analgesics freeze your pain, but they freeze up your bowels as well".

Is it causing other symptoms?
Severe constipation can cause colicky pain in the abdomen (which can radiate to the groin, chest and back) anorexia, malaise, nausea and vomiting and in the elderly confusion.

Is it causing "diarrhoea"?
Severe constipation can present as spurious diarrhoea, with small amounts of liquid faeces passing around the sides of a rectal bolus, often with some faecal incontinence.

Are faeces impacted?
It is important to do a rectal examination whenever it is suspected ("if you don't put your finger in you put your foot in"). In high constipation the rectum can be empty and ballooned. If there is doubt about the diagnosis a plain abdominal Xray will show faeces throughout the colon. For disimpaction give IM diamorphine 2.5mg (or more if on regular morphine) with midazolam 5–10mg, prior to the procedure.

How can it be prevented?
The best policy is aggressive prevention. Prescribe DAILY laxatives and start the same day as morphine or other opioid is started (eg Co-danthramer 20 ml nocte). The main aim of laxative use is an easy bowel action, not necessarily a daily one. Nevertheless it is a good idea to teach the patient the "3-day rule" – If the bowels are not open after 3 days a micro-enema or suppositories are needed (eg 5mg bisacodyl plus one glycerine suppository – which normally work within an hour).

Is there a contributory cause?
Common contributing factors (in addition to opioids) include dehydration, drugs (anti-cholinergics, vincristine, ondansetron) and difficulty getting access to a toilet or commode.

MODELS OF THE CONSULTATION

TRADITIONAL MODEL

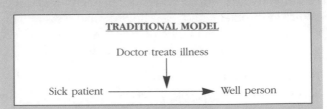

Doctor treats illness

Sick patient ──────────► Well person

BALINT'S MODEL (1957)

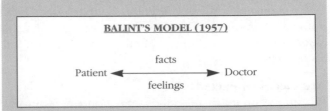

facts

Patient ◄──────────► Doctor

feelings

BYRNE AND LONG'S MODEL (1976)

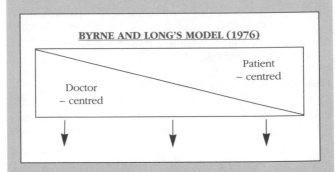

Patient
– centred

Doctor
– centred

PENDLETON'S MODEL (1984)

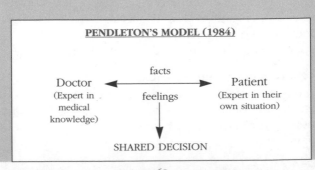

facts

Doctor ◄──────────► Patient
(Expert in   (Expert in their
medical   own situation)
knowledge)

feelings

SHARED DECISION

A consultation is when a person seeks advice from an expert. Advice is giving recommendations on appropriate choices of action.

The traditional model of the consultation assumed that if a doctor obtained enough information to make a diagnosis and then decide on treatment, the patient would be transformed back into a well person again. But this model didn't work for the majority of GP consultations, where the "illness" can't be defined and where 30% of complaints are psychological or psychosomatic. Nowadays it seems obvious that any consultation should involve shared decision-making with the patient, but this is a relatively new idea. In fact the consultation between a doctor and a patient has only been studied in recent years – mainly by GPs.

Balint's book "The Doctor, his Patient and the Illness" (1957) was a landmark because for the first time the consultation itself was analysed. The realisation that the feelings of both the doctor and the patient are involved now seems obvious. His group developed an approach, which they called "tuning in" – making contact with what is bothering the patient at that moment and simply checking out assumptions (rather than exploring feelings). His work led on to use of group discussions for GPs to analyse the emotional content of consultations for both the patient and themselves ("Balint groups").

Byrne & Long (1976) studied taped conversations between doctors and patients and found that patients are more likely to act on decisions if they have contributed to the decision-making process. After their work the term "patient-centred" became a byword for good practice, but in fact they found that a spectrum of styles is needed, and there can be a place for the doctor-centred approach to decision-making. (This is discussed in more detail in the section called Leadership.)

Pendleton's model (1984) stresses that patient's already have ideas, concerns and expectations about their illness (which can remain hidden) and these must be taken into consideration. I call it the "ICEberg theory" (because when an iceberg floats most of it is invisible below the surface) and I use it daily when making decisions with patients. This model also covers time:

I	=	**I**deas	=	The Past
C	=	**C**oncerns	=	The Present
E	=	**E**xpectations	=	The Future

Neighbour's Model (1987)

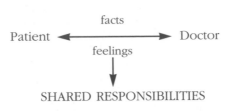

Patient ←→ facts →→ Doctor

feelings

SHARED RESPONSIBILITIES

Palliative Care Model – Linear

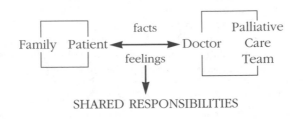

Family Patient ←→ facts →→ Doctor — Palliative Care Team

feelings

SHARED RESPONSIBILITIES

Palliative Care Model - Circular

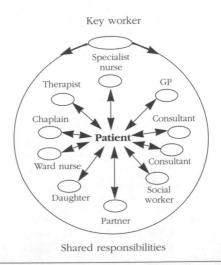

Key worker

Specialist nurse

Therapist   GP

Chaplain   Consultant

Patient

Ward nurse   Consultant

Daughter   Social worker

Partner

Shared responsibilities

Roger Neighbour's book "The Inner Consultation 1987" introduced the idea of "safety netting". He summarised his approach as:

1. Connecting with the patient
2. Summarising the problem
3. Handing over responsibility to the patient
4. Safety-netting
5. Housekeeping

Safety-netting means asking "What might happen if we have made the wrong decision?" It is a sharing of the uncertainties and the limits of knowledge with the patient, and is an ethical "safety net" for clinical decision-making.

The palliative care model of shared decision-making acknowledges the importance of both the family and the professional team and incorporates them into the model. It reminds us that any medical decision often sends ripples of concern around the patient's family. The diagram is linear, to show how the model has evolved from the doctor-patient consultation. However, the circular diagram underneath is a better representation of what really happens.

The circular model of palliative care shows how the patient is in the middle of a whole team of carers. The patient's decisions are often shaped by many mini-discussions with various professionals and relatives, who make up the caring team. The key worker, often a Macmillan nurse or District nurse, acts to facilitate communication between the team members by acting as an "and" in the system. This idea of being an "and" comes from a simple idea: for 1 and 1 to make 2, there has to be an "and" in the middle, to join them together. A team only functions if it is communicating together. The key worker decides who to involve for certain problems, and brings them together. This protects the patient from professional-overload. For example, to decide how to manage lymphoedema, the Macmillan nurse might arrange a meeting (to act as an "and") between the patient, the doctor and the physiotherapist, and that group may go on to make useful decisions, which any one person could not have made alone. The key worker might alert the patient to important decisions by asking previously unasked questions, eg "What do your children understand about your illness?" This model works well, but it requires "constructive gossiping" about the patient, and the dangers of breaking confidentiality or destructive gossiping are ever-present.

Is a team meeting needed?
By pooling information and generating new ideas a "group mind" can come up with better ideas than any one person. Team meetings can happen with or without the patient and relatives present.

What does the patient want?
Whenever a new decision is made on behalf of the patient, check it with the patient. Never talk to relatives without the patient's permission.

See Also: Family Meetings.

COUNSELLING

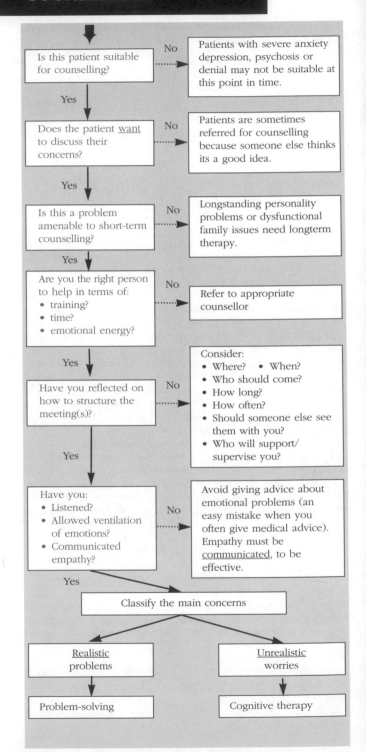

Is this patient suitable for counselling? → **No** → Patients with severe anxiety depression, psychosis or denial may not be suitable at this point in time.

↓ Yes

Does the patient <u>want</u> to discuss their concerns? → **No** → Patients are sometimes referred for counselling because someone else thinks its a good idea.

↓ Yes

Is this a problem amenable to short-term counselling? → **No** → Longstanding personality problems or dysfunctional family issues need longterm therapy.

↓ Yes

Are you the right person to help in terms of:
• training?
• time?
• emotional energy?
→ **No** → Refer to appropriate counsellor

↓ Yes

Have you reflected on how to structure the meeting(s)? → **No** → Consider:
• Where? • When?
• Who should come?
• How long?
• How often?
• Should someone else see them with you?
• Who will support/ supervise you?

↓ Yes

Have you:
• Listened?
• Allowed ventilation of emotions?
• Communicated empathy?
→ **No** → Avoid giving advice about emotional problems (an easy mistake when you often give medical advice). Empathy must be <u>communicated</u>, to be effective.

↓ Yes

Classify the main concerns

↙ ↘

<u>Realistic</u> problems → Problem-solving

<u>Unrealistic</u> worries → Cognitive therapy

When are counselling skills needed?

If the patient is unable to participate in decision making due to their emotional state they may well benefit from the use of counselling skills, to help them cope with their distress.

Am I the right person?

Anyone with warmth and common sense can listen to another person and encourage the open expression of feelings. If you have helped a person to talk and helped them listen to their own concerns and to feel differently – you have used counselling skills. <u>Note</u> that using "counselling skills" (which are needed in palliative care) is different to "counselling".

What is counselling?

Counselling is a therapeutic dialogue that occurs in the context of a framework agreed by a "contract" with a trained counsellor. It is intended to help a person change the way they feel and to become more self-confident and independent. If a patient becomes increasingly dependent it is not counselling (it is manipulation).The effectiveness of counselling depends on the personality and skill of the counsellor, who should be:

- encouraging (but calm)
- warm (but not possessive)
- empathic (but not manipulative)
- observant (but not judgmental)

Should the patient be referred to a counsellor?

A patient with complex emotional problems may need help from a trained counsellor. Counselling is on a spectrum of approaches which can be called "the talking cures".

APPROACH	AIM
Listening	Support
Counselling	Change feelings
Psychotherapy	Understand feelings (especially relating to childhood)
Psycho-analysis	Understand role of the unconscious in everyday life

A trained counsellor has an understanding of their own emotional needs, and has regular supervision (by another trained counsellor) because every one has vulnerabilities and emotional "blind spots."

Psychotherapy (to understand feelings) takes longer and is not usually appropriate to the palliative care setting, when time may be short, but a short course (eg 1 hour weekly, for 5 weeks) that is focused on specific aims can be very helpful (see Cognitive therapy).

See also Problem-solving and Cognitive therapy.

COUNSELLING COUPLES

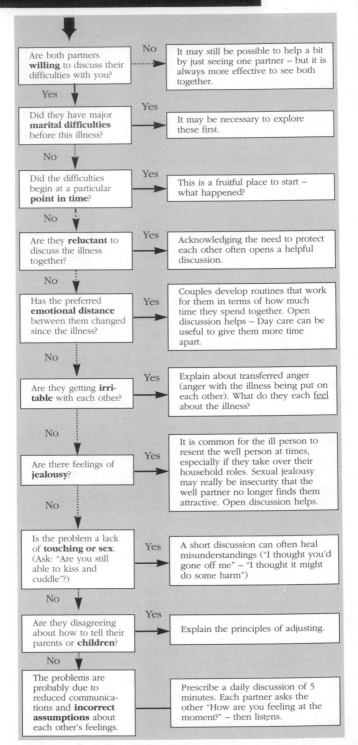

Are both partners **willing** to discuss their difficulties with you? → No → It may still be possible to help a bit by just seeing one partner – but it is always more effective to see both together.

↓ Yes

Did they have major **marital difficulties** before this illness? → Yes → It may be necessary to explore these first.

↓ No

Did the difficulties begin at a particular **point in time**? → Yes → This is a fruitful place to start – what happened?

↓ No

Are they **reluctant** to discuss the illness together? → Yes → Acknowledging the need to protect each other often opens a helpful discussion.

↓ No

Has the preferred **emotional distance** between them changed since the illness? → Yes → Couples develop routines that work for them in terms of how much time they spend together. Open discussion helps – Day care can be useful to give them more time apart.

↓ No

Are they getting **irritable** with each other? → Yes → Explain about transferred anger (anger with the illness being put on each other). What do they each <u>feel</u> about the illness?

↓ No

Are there feelings of **jealousy**? → Yes → It is common for the ill person to resent the well person at times, especially if they take over their household roles. Sexual jealousy may really be insecurity that the well partner no longer finds them attractive. Open discussion helps.

↓ No

Is the problem a lack of **touching or sex**. (Ask: "Are you still able to kiss and cuddle"?) → Yes → A short discussion can often heal misunderstandings ("I thought you'd gone off me" – "I thought it might do some harm")

↓ No

Are they disagreeing about how to tell their parents or **children**? → Yes → Explain the principles of adjusting.

↓ No

The problems are probably due to reduced communications and **incorrect assumptions** about each other's feelings. → Prescribe a daily discussion of 5 minutes. Each partner asks the other "How are you feeling at the moment?" – then listens.

Are the couple have difficulty communicating?

Illness tends to reduce communication between couples, because of tiredness, changed routines, worries about symptoms, medical appointments, increased family pressures, new relationships, loss of status, new roles, complex drug regimes, learning new skills (eg nursing), changes in the amount of time together, changes to personality or appearance and fears (going mad, pain, sudden unexpected death, being drugged). It is not surprising that communication suffers.

Are the difficulties long-standing?

A terminal illness can force a couple to accept that their disharmony is never going to improve and may lead to a major re-assessment of their relationship, and sometimes even a decision to separate. Formal help (from someone skilled in couple counselling (eg RELATE) may be needed as well.

Did the difficulties begin at a particular point in time?

This is a fruitful place to start. What happened? How did they feel? What are their assumptions about the effects on the other?

Are they trying to protect each other?

It may seem obvious and yet stating the obvious can open up a helpful discussion. Ask "How has this illness changed things for you both" – "How has it affected your relationship together?" Is there a fear that discussing practical issues (eg the will) may somehow make things worse?

Are they trying to protect others (children, parents)?

Emphasise that they know their family best, but also explain that everyone including children (from 2 upwards) cope best by knowing the truth, being allowed to ask questions and having time to adjust. Offer a family meeting.

Do they know what healthy conflict looks like?

Many couples benefit enormously from some simple explanation about how to communicate. Remind them that emotional maturity only happens through conflict.

HEALTHY CONFLICT FOR COUPLES

- **Verbalize feelings** ("I feel ... at the moment")
- **Take responsibility** for your own feelings ("I feel" NOT "You make me feel")
- **Avoid history** and be specific ("When X happened, I felt" NOT "You always ...")
- **Avoid mind-reading** (Ask "What did you feel ...?")
- **Avoid intellectual arguments** ("I feel" NOT "What you should do is ...")
- **Avoid non-verbal aggression** (sighs, silences etc)

CRISIS INTERVENTION

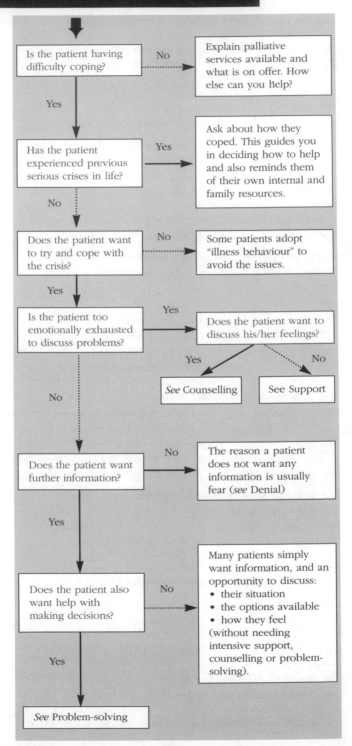

Is the patient having difficulty coping? → **No** → Explain palliative services available and what is on offer. How else can you help?

↓ **Yes**

Has the patient experienced previous serious crises in life? → **Yes** → Ask about how they coped. This guides you in deciding how to help and also reminds them of their own internal and family resources.

↓ **No**

Does the patient want to try and cope with the crisis? → **No** → Some patients adopt "illness behaviour" to avoid the issues.

↓ **Yes**

Is the patient too emotionally exhausted to discuss problems? → **Yes** → Does the patient want to discuss his/her feelings?

    Yes → *See* Counselling   **No** → See Support

↓ **No**

Does the patient want further information? → **No** → The reason a patient does not want any information is usually fear (*see* Denial)

↓ **Yes**

Does the patient also want help with making decisions? → **No** → Many patients simply want information, and an opportunity to discuss:
• their situation
• the options available
• how they feel (without needing intensive support, counselling or problem-solving).

↓ **Yes**

See Problem-solving

What is a crisis?

A crisis can be defined as an "temporary inability to cope with change". Palliative care is largely about trying to avoid crises (as far as possible) by discussion and planning. Nevertheless patients often <u>feel</u> like they are in a crisis. To solve a crisis decisions have to be made, but this can be difficult because a crisis causes both intellectual and emotional confusion.

What is crisis intervention?

Crisis intervention is a very useful model of care for understanding the role of palliative care professionals in helping patients. It focuses mainly on the need for decision-making, but assumes that a certain amount of emotional distress is inevitable as well.

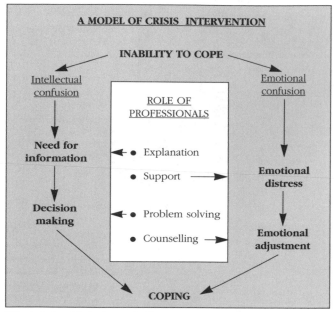

A MODEL OF CRISIS INTERVENTION

INABILITY TO COPE

Intellectual confusion → Need for information → Decision making

ROLE OF PROFESSIONALS
- Explanation
- Support
- Problem solving
- Counselling

Emotional confusion → Emotional distress → Emotional adjustment

COPING

What style of help is needed?

Professionals have to decide what style of help is most appropriate (explanation, support, problem-solving or counselling). Deciding on the appropriate style of help is important, because offering an inappropriate type of help will upset the patient:

eg   Offering nurturing support to a patient who only wants information ("Don't worry, we can worry about all that for you").

eg   Discussing detailed treatment options with a patient who is too emotionally distressed to take in any new information ("Which drug regime do you think you want?")

Usually a patient needs all 4 approaches but in differing degrees at different times (and this idea is discussed further in the section on Support).

See Also: Counselling, Explanation Problem-solving, Support and Transactional Analysis

DEATH CERTIFICATION

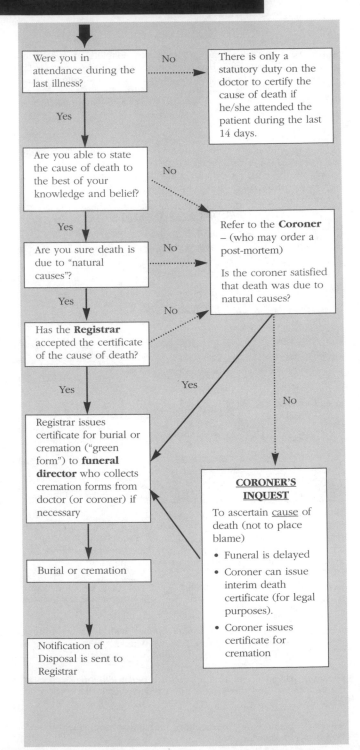

Were you in attendance during the last illness? → No → There is only a statutory duty on the doctor to certify the cause of death if he/she attended the patient during the last 14 days.

Yes ↓

Are you able to state the cause of death to the best of your knowledge and belief? → No

Yes ↓

Are you sure death is due to "natural causes"? → No

Yes ↓

Has the **Registrar** accepted the certificate of the cause of death? → No

Refer to the **Coroner** – (who may order a post-mortem)

Is the coroner satisfied that death was due to natural causes?

Yes / No

Yes ↓

Registrar issues certificate for burial or cremation ("green form") to **funeral director** who collects cremation forms from doctor (or coroner) if necessary

↓

Burial or cremation

↓

Notification of Disposal is sent to Registrar

CORONER'S INQUEST

To ascertain <u>cause</u> of death (not to place blame)

- Funeral is delayed
- Coroner can issue interim death certificate (for legal purposes).
- Coroner issues certificate for cremation

DEATH CERTIFICATION

What is the purpose of the death certificate?

Death certification started in 1837 to provide legal proof of death and to collect statistics about causes of death (hence the request on the certificate to know whether a post mortem is being held, in case further information about the cause of death is found – for epidemiological purposes).

What are the doctor's duties?

The doctor must issue a certificate of cause of death and has a legal responsibility to deliver the certificate to the Registrar of Births, Marriages and Deaths, (normally by asking a relative to deliver it as your agent, and giving them the "Notice to Informant" slip detached from the end of the certificate).

Did I see the patient within 14 days of death?

There is only a statutory duty on the doctor to certify the cause of death if he/she attended the patient during the last 14 days.

Do I know the cause of death?

Refer to the Coroner if the cause of death is unknown or where death may be due to an accident, self-neglect, suspicious circumstances, industrial disease, a surgical operation, or suicide.

The Coroner (or his deputy) is on call 24 hours a day. Most coroners are solicitors employed by the local Authority. The coroner's role is to establish the CAUSE of death. There is no legal duty on the doctor to report any death to the Coroner, but doctors are encouraged to report voluntarily any deaths that would need to be referred to the coroner by the registrar. If in doubt phone the coroner's officer for advice.

Have I completed the certificate correctly?

Give information about histology and site of cancer if possible eg "Cerebral metastases due to Squamous cell carcinoma of the left main bronchus" is better than "lung cancer".

If the certificate gives a *mode of death* rather than a cause (eg cardiac arrest, cardiac failure, coma, debility, liver failure, renal failure, respiratory arrest, shock), the registrar may decide to refer the death to the coroner if the certificate is not correctly completed (usually they phone to discuss it with the doctor first). If the certificate mentions the words "fracture" or "cirrhosis" the registrar is normally obliged to refer the death to the coroner.

Have I completed the cremation form and arranged for another doctor to complete part 2?

The regulations concerning cremation are more stringent because there are no traces of the body left for forensic purposes.

(*Note* – In Scotland the forms are different and the Procurator Fiscal is informed.)

DECISION ANALYSIS

DECISION TREE

This is a basic decision tree (ie without probabilities and utilities). A patient with advanced cancer of the bladder has become anaemic secondary to haemorrhage from the bladder, and the bleeding has now stopped. Should she have a blood transfusion?

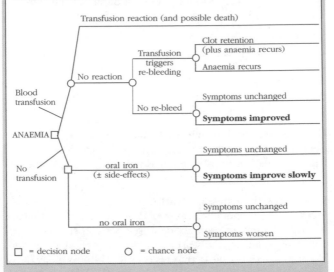

□ = decision node   ○ = chance node

PROBABILITIES

All possible outcomes are included so that probabilities at each node always add up to 1.

```
0.02           0.5           0.995
  ○              ○              ○
0.98           0.5           0.005
```

p = 1 = certain to occur
p = 0 = will never occur
p = 0.95 = 95% chance

UTILITIES

Probability	Outcome	Utility (preference)
0.25	re-bleed	0.05
0.75	no re-bleed	0.95

1 = Optimum outcome (100% utility)
0 = least preferred option
0.95 = 95% utility

The weighted utility for a re-bleed (0.05 × 0.25 = 0.0125) will make transfusion an unlikely option for this patient.

PROBABILITIES

The decision will be affected by **probabilities**. For example the probability of a transfusion reaction is generally low, say 0.005 (5 per 1000 or 1 in 200). But if a patient has had a previous transfusion reaction, the probability (risk, chance) may be a lot higher. Unfortunately probabilities in medicine (and especially in palliative medicine) are often not known, and a "best guess" estimate has to be made from a combination of experience and observational studies.

WEIGHTED UTILITIES

The decision will be also affected by the patient's **preferences** (known as "utilities" in decision analysis). Each outcome is give as a utility score (0–1) and the preferred course of action can be be calculated by considering the "weighted utility" (probability × utility) for each option. The weighted utility of 2 branches can be added together to give a score for the previous decision point, and these can be added as well, to give a score for the previous decision. The branch with the highest weighted utility score is the best course of action for that patient.

DECISION ANALYSIS

What is decision analysis?
Decision analysis is a systematic method of identifying possible courses of action and then assessing the probability and utility (usefulness to the patient) of each outcome and then calculating the optimal course of action.

Decisions analysis has been widely used in business for years. In medicine it is rarely used for individual patient care and more often used to shed light on important medical controversies e.g. the best management for ovarian cancer (*Simes* 1985). Decision analysis can guide clinical decisions by considering the two uncertainties,

a) Probabilities
b) Patient preferences (utility)

In reality *probabilities* and *preference* values often remain uncertain, but at least decision analysis makes these uncertainties explicit.

Where is decision analysis useful?
Decision analysis is not necessary if a wrong decision is unimportant or if the correct course of action is obvious to everyone. But it is useful in complex decisions. It assumes that all possible courses of action can be identified and these are then represented in a decision tree consisting of the starting point, various alternatives, probable events and outcomes. The best course of action is the one with the highest weighted utility.

It can still be useful to draw a decision tree even if the definite probabilities are not known, because it is impossible to keep several facets of a decision in the mind simultaneously and analysis of a problem by intuition alone can make major simplifying assumptions.

What about the cost of treatments?
Decision analysis can be useful in policy-making to reconcile evidence based medicine with patient preferences and health economics.

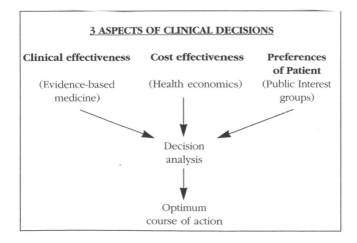

3 ASPECTS OF CLINICAL DECISIONS

Clinical effectiveness   **Cost effectiveness**   **Preferences of Patient**

(Evidence-based medicine)   (Health economics)   (Public Interest groups)

Decision analysis

Optimum course of action

DECISION MAKING I
– A model

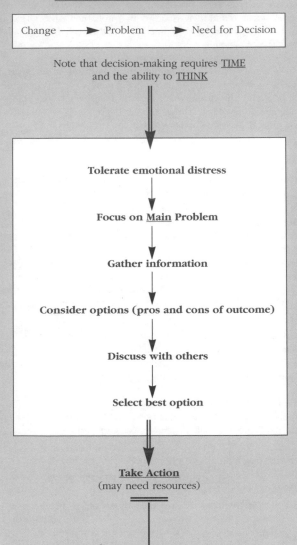

A MODEL OF DECISION-MAKING

Change ──────▶ Problem ──────▶ Need for Decision

Note that decision-making requires <u>TIME</u>
and the ability to <u>THINK</u>

Tolerate emotional distress

Focus on <u>Main</u> Problem

Gather information

Consider options (pros and cons of outcome)

Discuss with others

Select best option

<u>**Take Action**</u>
(may need resources)

IS ANYTHING PREVENTING ACTION OCCURRING?

- Lack of Resources (training, equipment)
- Lack of authority over others
- Disputes
- Ambivalence
- No forum for discussion

What is Decision-making?

Decision-making means selecting a course of action to solve a specific problem. All behaviour involves simple decisions. It can be important to ask: "what happens if I do nothing?". A decision is <u>important</u> if the cost of failing to achieve the objective is high. A decision is <u>urgent</u> if the cost of failing increases with time. (Notice that all the "steps" in the model opposite may happen simultaneously).

Is a decision needed?

Decision-making is not necessary if:

  – the best course of action is clear to everyone
  – there is only one option
  – the patient has no preferences
  – no possible action would make a difference
  – the consequences of a wrong decision are unimportant

Can the patient think?

Is the patient too exhausted to think about the problem at the moment? Is the patient mentally competent to make the decision? (see Consent).

Is time needed?

Some decisions can be anticipated, which allows more time for data gathering and discussion. Anticipation may have to be initiated by asking hypothetical questions, eg "IF the time comes for you to need more nursing help, where would you like to be looked after?"

Does the patient need help coping with emotional distress?

The patient may not be in a state to make decisions, and may need support or counselling (see Crisis Intervention). The patient may have regressed emotionally and may want others to make the decisions for them (see Transactional analysis).

What is the main problem?

"The art of medicine remains the art of identifying the patient's problem, which is something more than merely diagnosing his disease."

Robert Platt

Is information needed?

Patients need information in an understandable form (see Information). The patient may feel unable to cope with the information (see Denial). Doctors need two sorts of information: 1 about the patient's medical history, 2 about the particular disease process.

Is discussion needed?

Many patients want a "therapeutic dialogue", to understand information, or to relate it to their own situation. (Some patients request a second opinion not because they are dissatisfied with a doctor but because it is easier to understand a problem if more than one perspective is taken.) Patients often need to have a discussion with friends and family, to consider the opinions of others, before making important decisions.

Does the patient need help choosing between various options?

The patient may benefit from learning about different ways of choosing between options (see Decision-making 3 and Problem-solving).

DECISION MAKING II
– Ways of deciding

WAYS OF MAKING DECISIONS	
Research-based	Provides quick access to experience of others but may not be appropriate to a particular situation or decision. Limited by scarcity of research.
Pros and Cons	A simple way of taking many factors into account, but assumes all the points have equal importance (see Problem-Solving).
Ranking of options	Make a list of some important criteria that each option should meet. Then see which option fulfils the most criteria. These can be scored so that the most important criteria contributes more to the decision ("weighted ranking").
Hurdles	Eliminate options by setting successively sterner hurdles. Good for choosing between very varied options. The hurdles may relate to: • cost • time needed • disturbance to routines • inconvenience to others, etc
Clustering	Deals with a large number of ideas or options by clustering them into groups, then choosing between the groups (eg by using pros and cons of each group). Groups may need re-configuring to combine best options together.
Intuition	The choice of option is based on which feels best. Decisions based on intuition may be biased by emotions or prejudice. Appropriate if other information is lacking (see Internal factors).
Voting	Each person votes for one option. Democratic. Assumes the views of each person are of equal importance.
Consensus	A group of people discuss a problem and come to a combined (or modified or compromise) decision. Time-consuming, but increases the commitment of each person to the decision (eg patient, relatives and carers discussing a discharge plan – see Discharge planning).

How is the best option selected?

In order to make a choice the patient needs to work through in his or her mind the implications of each option. A good way of doing this is to consider the pros and cons of each option, and this is discussed in more detail in the section on Problem Solving.

What will the consequences be?

Some options will have outcomes that are more predictable than others. The role of the professional is often to help the patient try to explore the consequences of their decision.

Can criteria be identified that the best option should meet?

If the patient can list some criteria that they would like the best option to meet it can help in identifying their best option. For example in choosing a treatment option they may have certain criteria in their mind, and it can help if these are made known to the team. For example, the criteria that the best option should meet may be:

- Does not involve a surgical operation
- Easy to manage at home
- Very low risk of causing nausea
- No injections needed
- Likely to control symptoms

Can the criteria be put in order of preference?

The criteria can be given a score, or ranking, so that the most important criteria contribute more to the decision. For example if a patient was especially concerned that a treatment would be easy to manage at home, then this criteria could be ranked 1 or given the most number of points. Another patient who was needle-phobic might rank the "no injections" criteria very highly.

Do you agree with the patient's choice?

You may need to check your own attitude. The patient may make a decision that is different to the one you would make. You must remain impartial and give information in a non-judgmental way. Avoid the temptation of influencing them to make the choice that is easier for you to organize.

Is the patient having trouble deciding?

The patient may need time to reflect or to ask more questions ("you do not have to decide right away") and should be encouraged to discuss the decision with family or close friends. Some patients need affirmation that they are allowed to assert their own choice.

See Also: Problem Solving

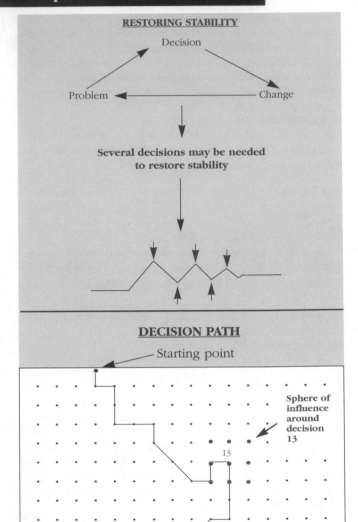

RESTORING STABILITY

Decision

Problem ← → Change

**Several decisions may be needed
to restore stability**

DECISION PATH

Starting point

Sphere of influence around decision 13

13

End point

Each change leads to new influences, which cannot be clearly predicted, so the decisions to be taken cannot be predicted. Note there are many different potential decision paths to the same final end points

What happens if the decision is wrong?

Decisions are often wrong or partially wrong. A problem often requires several decisions, in order to restore stability. Decision-making is often a process, rather than a single event, which gradually restores stability. Each decision leads to change, which may produce another problem, requiring another decision (represented by the wavy line at the bottom of the top diagram).

In what order should decisions be made?

The more things you can do, the more complex it gets. If you only have 2 things you can do, there are only 2 orders to do them in. But if there are 5 things you need to do, there are 120 possible sequences for doing them. For example a patient may need antibiotics, radiotherapy, surgery and anti-coagulation. What is the logical order? Which is most urgent? Will doing one thing make the next one more difficult? The puzzle below is a good example of the importance (and the difficulty) of considering the logical order of making decisions.

A PUZZLE

A man with a small boat needs to transport a fox, a chicken and some grain across a river. He can only take them across one at a time. Given the chance the fox would eat the chicken, and the chicken would eat the grain – therefore these pairs cannot be left alone together. Which order does the man take them across? (eg he can't take the fox first because then the chicken would eat the grain). How does he do it?

What other factors influence decisions?

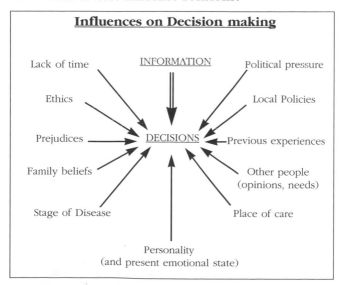

Influences on Decision making

Lack of time

INFORMATION

Political pressure

Ethics

Local Policies

Prejudices — DECISIONS ←— Previous experiences

Family beliefs

Other people
(opinions, needs)

Stage of Disease

Place of care

Personality
(and present emotional state)

DECISION-MAKING IV
– clinical decisions

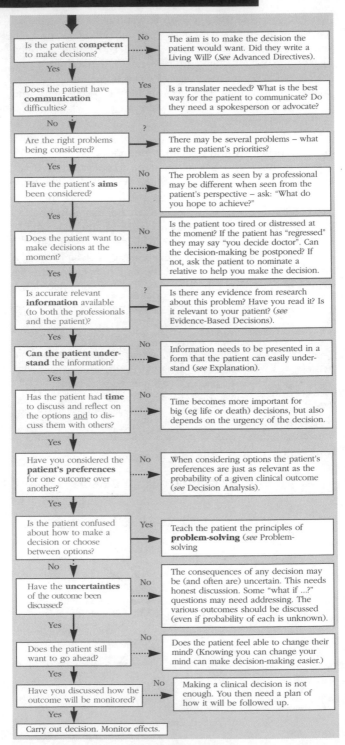

Is the patient competent to make decisions? — No → The aim is to make the decision the patient would want. Did they write a Living Will? (*See* Advanced Directives).

Yes ↓

Does the patient have communication difficulties? — Yes → Is a translator needed? What is the best way for the patient to communicate? Do they need a spokesperson or advocate?

No ↓

Are the right problems being considered? — ? → There may be several problems – what are the patient's priorities?

Yes ↓

Have the patient's aims been considered? — No → The problem as seen by a professional may be different when seen from the patient's perspective – ask: "What do you hope to achieve?"

Yes ↓

Does the patient want to make decisions at the moment? — No → Is the patient too tired or distressed at the moment? If the patient has "regressed" they may say "you decide doctor". Can the decision-making be postponed? If not, ask the patient to nominate a relative to help you make the decision.

Yes ↓

Is accurate relevant information available (to both the professionals and the patient)? — ? → Is there any evidence from research about this problem? Have you read it? Is it relevant to your patient? (*see* Evidence-Based Decisions).

Yes ↓

Can the patient understand the information? — No → Information needs to be presented in a form that the patient can easily understand (*see* Explanation).

Yes ↓

Has the patient had time to discuss and reflect on the options <u>and</u> to discuss them with others? — No → Time becomes more important for big (eg life or death) decisions, but also depends on the urgency of the decision.

Yes ↓

Have you considered the patient's preferences for one outcome over another? — No → When considering options the patient's preferences are just as relevant as the probability of a given clinical outcome (*see* Decision Analysis).

Yes ↓

Is the patient confused about how to make a decision or choose between options? — Yes → Teach the patient the principles of **problem-solving** (*see* Problem-solving

No ↓

Have the uncertainties of the outcome been discussed? — No → The consequences of any decision may be (and often are) uncertain. This needs honest discussion. Some "what if ...?" questions may need addressing. The various outcomes should be discussed (even if probability of each is unknown).

Yes ↓

Does the patient still want to go ahead? — No → Does the patient feel able to change their mind? (Knowing you can change your mind can make decision-making easier.)

Yes ↓

Have you discussed how the outcome will be monitored? — No → Making a clinical decision is not enough. You then need a plan of how it will be followed up.

Yes ↓

Carry out decision. Monitor effects.

Does the patient have a goal?

The patient may be confused about what their goal is, but if no goal exists the patient has no preferences for different options, then decision-making is unnecessary. Goals should be **SMART** (Specific, Measurable, Achievable, Realistic and Timed (eg short-term).

Can the patient think?

If the patient is emotionally distressed (due to fear, anger, guilt or sadness) it makes it difficult or impossible to think clearly enough to make important decisions. It may be necessary to deal with emotional distress before focusing on the decision-making (*see* Crisis intervention and Counselling).

Does the patient have accurate information?

To make decisions a person needs information. What is the quality of information? Has it been explained clearly? Does the patient understand it? Does the patient want to verify it? Does it need to be given in written as well as verbal form?.

Does the patient need a dialogue with an expert?

When making any decision we need to consider the advantages and disadvantages of the various options. When making medical decisions emotional and social factors may be very important to the patient. Decision-making therefore needs to be shared between the patient and the professional.

Is there enough time to reflect?

The patient may want to seek the opinion of family and friends to consider further options before making an important decision, or may want further information and explanation. Time may not be available (see Emergencies).

How much support does the patient want?

It can be very helpful to ask the patient "Are you the sort of person who likes to make decisions or are you the sort of person who likes to leave it to other people or are you somewhere in between?" Patient's in a crisis sometimes regress to being emotionally dependent and they may want quite a lot of guidance.

Has change happened?

Who has the power to make things happen? Is someone blocking the changes? The aim is to restore stability, but the decisions may be wrong or may lead to other problems. Stability may be only restored gradually over a period of time and after a series of related decisions.

See also: Consent, Ethical problems

DEHYDRATION

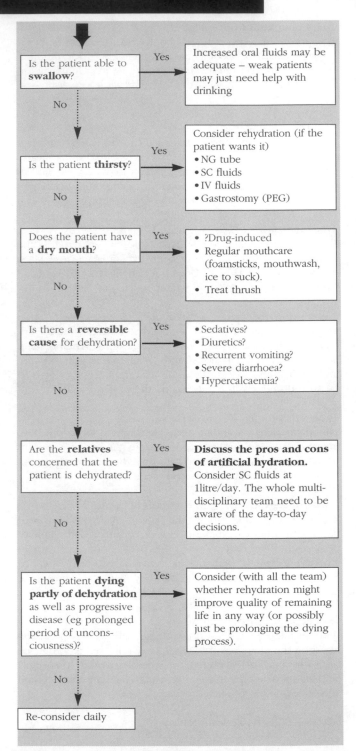

Is the patient able to **swallow**?

Yes → Increased oral fluids may be adequate – weak patients may just need help with drinking

No ↓

Is the patient **thirsty**?

Yes → Consider rehydration (if the patient wants it)
- NG tube
- SC fluids
- IV fluids
- Gastrostomy (PEG)

No ↓

Does the patient have a **dry mouth**?

Yes →
- ?Drug-induced
- Regular mouthcare (foamsticks, mouthwash, ice to suck).
- Treat thrush

No ↓

Is there a **reversible cause** for dehydration?

Yes →
- Sedatives?
- Diuretics?
- Recurrent vomiting?
- Severe diarrhoea?
- Hypercalcaemia?

No ↓

Are the **relatives** concerned that the patient is dehydrated?

Yes → **Discuss the pros and cons of artificial hydration.** Consider SC fluids at 1litre/day. The whole multi-disciplinary team need to be aware of the day-to-day decisions.

No ↓

Is the patient **dying partly of dehydration** as well as progressive disease (eg prolonged period of unconsciousness)?

Yes → Consider (with all the team) whether rehydration might improve quality of remaining life in any way (or possibly just be prolonging the dying process).

No ↓

Re-consider daily

90

Is the patient dehydrated?

Dry tongue, sunken eyes, inelastic skin, fast pulse, poor urine output (and dark urine) all suggest dehydration. Sodium urea and albumin levels may be elevated. The patient may not be thirsty.

Is re-hydration indicated?

Towards death, a person's desire for food and drink lessens. Artificial hydration does not normally improve comfort or survival. IV re-hydration is usually indicated if there is a possibility of a potentially correctable cause (eg excessive diuretics, sedation, recurrent vomiting, diarrhoea or hypercalcaemia).

Is a dry mouth the main problem?

Some dehydration commonly occurs when a dying patient becomes too weak to swallow. Dry mouth is common but responds to good mouth care (reassess any medication that may be contributing to it). Artificial hydration is unnecessary just for dry mouth

Is the patient thirsty?

If the patient is thirsty they should be re-hydrated, orally if possible. Hydration of semi-conscious patients in the hospice or nursing home setting is easier to achieve now that the subcutaneous route has become commonly used for fluid, (eg 1 litre of normal saline or 5% glucose per 12-24 hours by SC infusion – usually in the thigh or abdomen). 3l per day can be infused if necessary by using 2 sites. 1500 units of hyaluronidase (Hyalase) is sometimes used to prime the line to help the fluid diffuse into the subcutaneous tissues – but it is not essential.

Should a hospice have a policy about re-hydration?

No. The appropriateness of artificial hydration continues to depend on regular assessment of the likely benefits and burdens of such intervention. A blanket policy of either always giving artificial hydration, or of no artificial hydration, is ethically indefensible. The appropriateness of artificial hydration for a patient should be judged on a day-to-day basis, weighing up the potential harms and benefits. The decisions should involve the multi-professional team, the patient, and relatives and carers, but the senior doctor has ultimate responsibility for the decision. A competent patient has the right to refuse artificial hydration, even if it is considered of clinical benefit. Incompetent patients retain this right through a valid advance refusal (*see* Living Wills).

See also: Terminal phase

DENIAL

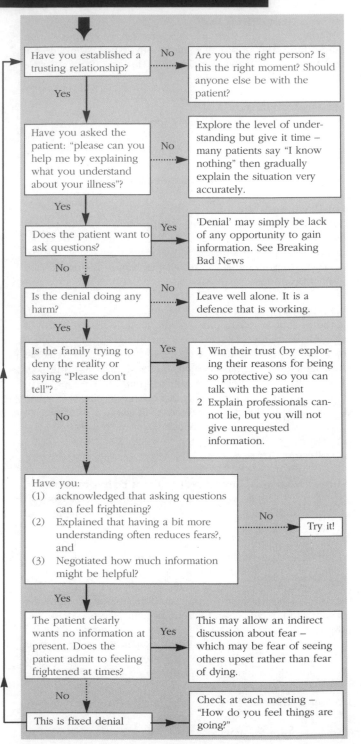

Have you established a trusting relationship? —No→ Are you the right person? Is this the right moment? Should anyone else be with the patient?

↓ Yes

Have you asked the patient: "please can you help me by explaining what you understand about your illness"? —No→ Explore the level of understanding but give it time – many patients say "I know nothing" then gradually explain the situation very accurately.

↓ Yes

Does the patient want to ask questions? —Yes→ 'Denial' may simply be lack of any opportunity to gain information. See Breaking Bad News

↓ No

Is the denial doing any harm? —No→ Leave well alone. It is a defence that is working.

↓ Yes

Is the family trying to deny the reality or saying "Please don't tell"? —Yes→ 1 Win their trust (by exploring their reasons for being so protective) so you can talk with the patient
2 Explain professionals cannot lie, but you will not give unrequested information.

↓ No

Have you:
(1) acknowledged that asking questions can feel frightening?
(2) Explained that having a bit more understanding often reduces fears?, and
(3) Negotiated how much information might be helpful? —No→ Try it!

↓ Yes

The patient clearly wants no information at present. Does the patient admit to feeling frightened at times? —Yes→ This may allow an indirect discussion about fear – which may be fear of seeing others upset rather than fear of dying.

↓ No

This is fixed denial —→ Check at each meeting – "How do you feel things are going?"

92

What is denial?
Denial regulates the rate at which a person has to face painful information, and most patients use denial from time to time to help them cope. Denial is a normal psychological defence (related to selective attention, which we all use every day).

Is the patient in denial?
Find out what he/she knows, or wants to know. Patients may be open with some people but not others. Patients may deny at some times and be more accepting at others. As a patient begins to feel more safe and secure and trusting they usually begin to face up to the reality, little by little. Fixed denial that does not change is very rare.

Is the denial doing any harm?
If denial is not causing any problems there is no need to challenge it. However excessive denial can cause anxiety and can make family communication very difficult.

Nightmares or panic attacks may also occur in patients in total fixed denial.

Should the denial be challenged?
Never give unrequested information which simply causes anxiety or anger. Fixed denial can only be challenged in the context of a relationship of mutual trust. Ask: "How do you feel things are going at the moment". The patient must feel safe in order to ask questions. If they want to ask questions, go gently (see Breaking Bad News). Note that if the patient begins addressing denial and facing reality it reduces fear but tends to increase sadness for a time.

Do you find the patient's denial uncomfortable?
Denial in a patient can feel uncomfortable, (because you are being invited to take part in an unrealistic fantasy.) However, it is not always appropriate to challenge denial, in which case it is still possible to be positive without being untruthful, eg

patient: I'm sure I'm getting better
doctor: That's good – I hope you soon feel better. Are there any questions you want to ask me at the moment?
patient: Not really – no.

Is the family in denial?
Family denial is distressing because everyone fears saying the wrong thing and communication suffers. The aim is to work step-by-step towards a conversation with the patient and family together in which they are all at the same level of understanding.

Does the patient admit to feeling frightened at times?
If the patient agrees to feeling afraid, it opens doors to look at the reasons for the fear. Ask: "What was happening at the time?" (and the feelings emerge) and then ask: "What do you think the fears might be about?" Ask about the details of any nightmares because describing and verbalizing fears helps – and it feels safer to discuss fearful feelings due to a dream rather than due to the illness itself.

DEPRESSION

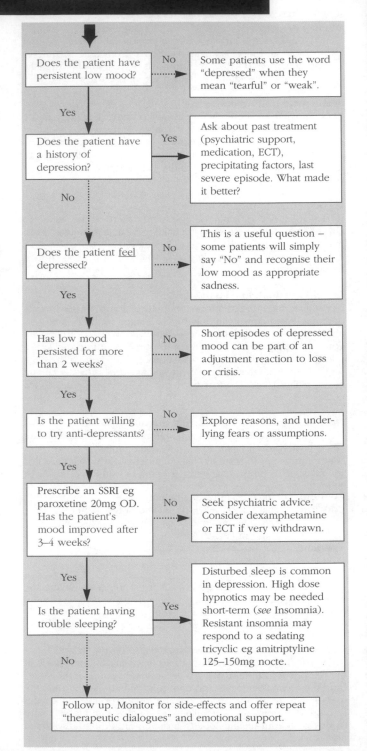

Does the patient have persistent low mood? — No → Some patients use the word "depressed" when they mean "tearful" or "weak".

Yes ↓

Does the patient have a history of depression? — Yes → Ask about past treatment (psychiatric support, medication, ECT), precipitating factors, last severe episode. What made it better?

No ↓

Does the patient <u>feel</u> depressed? — No → This is a useful question – some patients will simply say "No" and recognise their low mood as appropriate sadness.

Yes ↓

Has low mood persisted for more than 2 weeks? — No → Short episodes of depressed mood can be part of an adjustment reaction to loss or crisis.

Yes ↓

Is the patient willing to try anti-depressants? — No → Explore reasons, and underlying fears or assumptions.

Yes ↓

Prescribe an SSRI eg paroxetine 20mg OD. Has the patient's mood improved after 3–4 weeks? — No → Seek psychiatric advice. Consider dexamphetamine or ECT if very withdrawn.

Yes ↓

Is the patient having trouble sleeping? — Yes → Disturbed sleep is common in depression. High dose hypnotics may be needed short-term (*see* Insomnia). Resistant insomnia may respond to a sedating tricyclic eg amitriptyline 125–150mg nocte.

No ↓

Follow up. Monitor for side-effects and offer repeat "therapeutic dialogues" and emotional support.

Is it depression?
Sometimes patients will label themselves as "depressed" when they mean they had an episode of tearfulness or feel disappointed about being weaker. It can be very helpful (and useful for patients) if we distinguish between 3 separate experiences (which may overlap):

- Appropriate sadness (grief)
- Adjustment reaction (crisis)
- Clinical depression (persistent low mood).

Is it appropriate sadness?
Being ill or dying involves a whole series of losses (eg loss of independence, loss of driving, loss of role). Grief is different to depression. People with a history of depression, who then experience grief, say grief feels less unpleasant, because it is possible to work at it. Help the person talk of the loss, what it means and how they feel about it. This helps them to begin to adjust emotionally, and to re-invest their emotions elsewhere.

Is it part of an adjustment reaction?
Overcoming the "emotional storm" of a crisis (see Crisis Intervention) takes 1–2 weeks for most patients. They may need intensive support short-term (see Counselling), and practical adjustments may be needed (see Problem Solving).

Is it clinical depression?
The key features are constant low mood (lasting longer than 2 weeks), low self-esteem and inability to smile or enjoy anything. It may progress to paranoia, delusions or agitation. Anti-depressants plus emotional support and counselling are more effective than either one alone.

What about resistant depression?
10–15% of patients will not respond to first line anti-depressants. Treatments for resistant depression include increasing the dose, using broad spectrum SNRI drugs which act at both 5HT and noradrenergic receptors (eg clomipramine, venlafaxine) measuring TCA levels, considering anti-psychotic therapy. or adding Lithium (which augments the action of both 5HT and NA anti-depressants.) 50% of patients starting Lithium will improve after 3 weeks. Combinations of TCA, SSRI and Lithium can be given. Alternatively MAOI with Lithium can be used. ECT can still have a place in advanced cancer if the patient is profoundly withdrawn, and has an effect in 2-3 days. These treatments need to be supervised by a Psychiatrist.

DETERIORATION

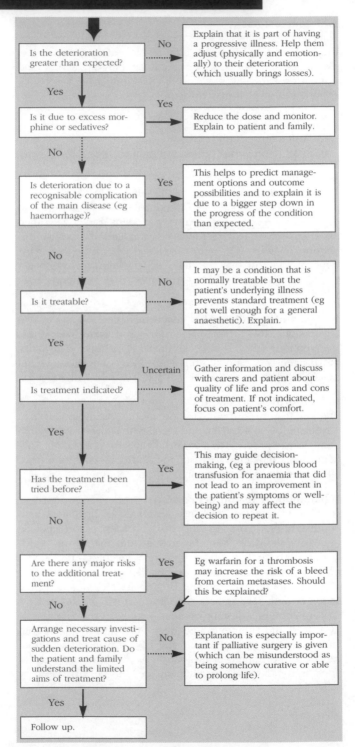

Is the deterioration greater than expected?
→ No → Explain that it is part of having a progressive illness. Help them adjust (physically and emotionally) to their deterioration (which usually brings losses).

↓ Yes

Is it due to excess morphine or sedatives?
→ Yes → Reduce the dose and monitor. Explain to patient and family.

↓ No

Is deterioration due to a recognisable complication of the main disease (eg haemorrhage)?
→ Yes → This helps to predict management options and outcome possibilities and to explain it is due to a bigger step down in the progress of the condition than expected.

↓ No

Is it treatable?
→ No → It may be a condition that is normally treatable but the patient's underlying illness prevents standard treatment (eg not well enough for a general anaesthetic). Explain.

↓ Yes

Is treatment indicated?
→ Uncertain → Gather information and discuss with carers and patient about quality of life and pros and cons of treatment. If not indicated, focus on patient's comfort.

↓ Yes

Has the treatment been tried before?
→ Yes → This may guide decision-making, (eg a previous blood transfusion for anaemia that did not lead to an improvement in the patient's symptoms or well-being) and may affect the decision to repeat it.

↓ No

Are there any major risks to the additional treatment?
→ Yes → Eg warfarin for a thrombosis may increase the risk of a bleed from certain metastases. Should this be explained?

↓ No

Arrange necessary investigations and treat cause of sudden deterioration. Do the patient and family understand the limited aims of treatment?
→ No → Explanation is especially important if palliative surgery is given (which can be misunderstood as being somehow curative or able to prolong life).

↓ Yes

Follow up.

Is deterioration due to the underlying disease?

If deterioration is due to the expected progression of the disease it can be very helpful simply to state this, because it may <u>not</u> be obvious to the patient and relatives. Explanation that the problem is part of the same condition (and not due to yet another illness) can be helpful.

Is deterioration happening at the expected rate?

Sudden deterioration may be due to the underlying cancer, but treatable complications (such as metabolic disturbances, emboli or infection) should be excluded.

Is deterioration following an unusual pattern?

It can be very confusing where deterioration follows an unusual pattern. For example a patient with brain metastases who was deteriorating week by week, suddenly became unconscious and was thought to be dying. However she gradually started to recover, which made the relatives over-optimistic. In fact the patient had had an acute CVA in addition to brain metastases which had complicated the usual pattern of step-by-step deterioration from brain metastases and made it difficult for the relatives to understand what was happening.

Is deterioration happening every day?

Daily deterioration in a patient with advanced cancer in the absence of any explanations such as infection usually means the patient is entering the terminal phase of the illness and only has a few days to live.

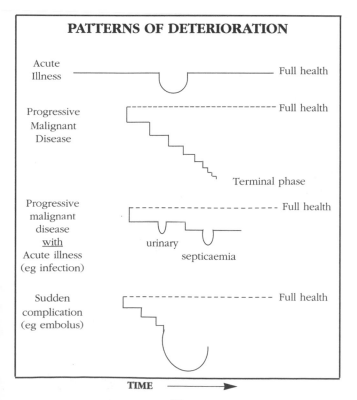

PATTERNS OF DETERIORATION

Acute Illness — Full health

Progressive Malignant Disease — Full health / Terminal phase

Progressive malignant disease <u>with</u> Acute illness (eg infection) — Full health / urinary septicaemia

Sudden complication (eg embolus) — Full health

TIME ⟶

DIARRHOEA

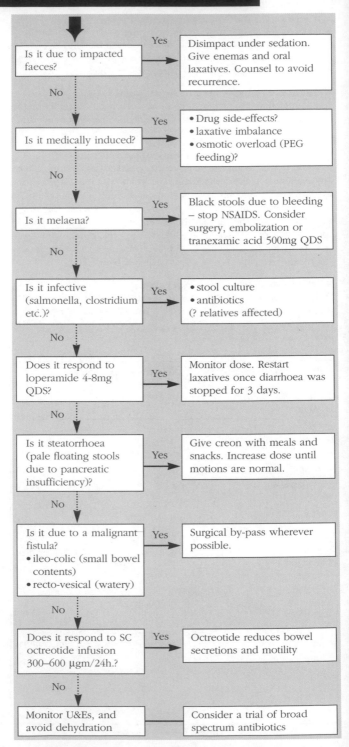

Is it due to impacted faeces?

Yes → Disimpact under sedation. Give enemas and oral laxatives. Counsel to avoid recurrence.

No

Is it medically induced?

Yes →
- Drug side-effects?
- laxative imbalance
- osmotic overload (PEG feeding)?

No

Is it melaena?

Yes → Black stools due to bleeding – stop NSAIDS. Consider surgery, embolization or tranexamic acid 500mg QDS

No

Is it infective (salmonella, clostridium etc.)?

Yes →
- stool culture
- antibiotics
(? relatives affected)

No

Does it respond to loperamide 4-8mg QDS?

Yes → Monitor dose. Restart laxatives once diarrhoea was stopped for 3 days.

No

Is it steatorrhoea (pale floating stools due to pancreatic insufficiency)?

Yes → Give creon with meals and snacks. Increase dose until motions are normal.

No

Is it due to a malignant fistula?
- ileo-colic (small bowel contents)
- recto-vesical (watery)

Yes → Surgical by-pass wherever possible.

No

Does it respond to SC octreotide infusion 300–600 µgm/24h.?

Yes → Octreotide reduces bowel secretions and motility

No

Monitor U&Es, and avoid dehydration — Consider a trial of broad spectrum antibiotics

Is it due to impacted faeces?

This is the commonest cause of diarrhoea in the hospice setting. Small amounts of liquid motion (sometimes with incontinence) suggest overflow past an impacted lump of faeces in the rectum. There is a history of severe constipation before the diarrhoea started. Digital evacuation is needed, then education about the use of laxatives.

Is it due to excess laxatives?

Patients commonly get into a cycle of laxative misuse (getting a bit constipated, taking too much laxative, having diarrhoea, stopping the laxatives, getting constipated). Teach regular daily use of laxatives. Diarrhoea may be also a side-effect of other drugs (eg antibiotics).

Is it melaena?

Black tarry stools suggests bleeding higher up the bowel. Test for blood and check the Hb level. Blood transfusion is only indicated if the bleeding can be controlled.<None>

Is it infective?

Sudden onset of diarrhoea and vomiting together strongly suggests gastro-enteritis is the cause. Have others been affected? Send stool cultures and take advice from the bacteriologist about treatment.

Is it malabsorbtion?

Cancer of the pancreas (and sometimes other upper abdominal malignancies) can cause obstruction to the pancreatic duct and malabsorbtion of fat causing frequent smelly pale motions that tend to float. Loperamide is ineffective but it responds well to pancreatic enzyme therapy such as creon (1–3 with meals and 1 with snacks or milky drinks).

Is it due to a fistula?

Persistent diarrhoea in a patient with intra-abdominal malignancy suggests a fistula may have occurred. A fistula from the small bowel into the colon causes undigested small bowel contents to pass very rapidly through the bowel. If surgical repair is not an option treat with octreotide.

Is it severe enough to cause dehydration?

Check U&Es and consider rehydration. Chronic diarrhoea can cause low potassium levels.

DISCHARGE PLANNING

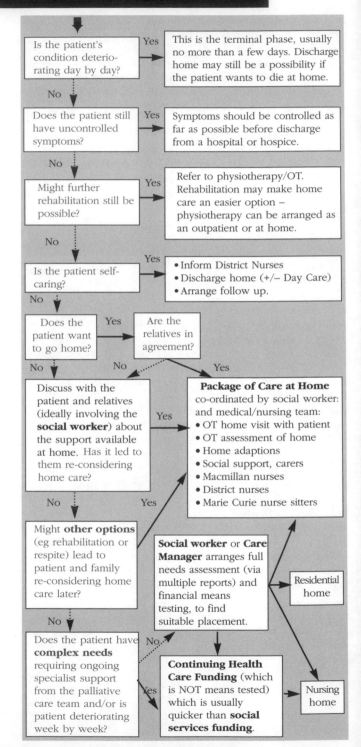

Is the patient's condition deteriorating day by day? — Yes → This is the terminal phase, usually no more than a few days. Discharge home may still be a possibility if the patient wants to die at home.

No ↓

Does the patient still have uncontrolled symptoms? — Yes → Symptoms should be controlled as far as possible before discharge from a hospital or hospice.

No ↓

Might further rehabilitation still be possible? — Yes → Refer to physiotherapy/OT. Rehabilitation may make home care an easier option – physiotherapy can be arranged as an outpatient or at home.

No ↓

Is the patient self-caring? — Yes →
• Inform District Nurses
• Discharge home (+/– Day Care)
• Arrange follow up.

No ↓

Does the patient want to go home? — Yes → **Are the relatives in agreement?**

No ↓   No ↘   Yes ↓

Discuss with the patient and relatives (ideally involving the **social worker**) about the support available at home. Has it led to them re-considering home care? — Yes →

Package of Care at Home co-ordinated by social worker: and medical/nursing team:
• OT home visit with patient
• OT assessment of home
• Home adaptions
• Social support, carers
• Macmillan nurses
• District nurses
• Marie Curie nurse sitters

No ↓

Might **other options** (eg rehabilitation or respite) lead to patient and family re-considering home care later? — Yes ↗

Social worker or **Care Manager** arranges full needs assessment (via multiple reports) and financial means testing, to find suitable placement. → Residential home

No ↓

Does the patient have **complex needs** requiring ongoing specialist support from the palliative care team and/or is patient deteriorating week by week? — No ↖

Yes ↓

Continuing Health Care Funding (which is NOT means tested) which is usually quicker than **social services funding**. → Nursing home

DISCHARGE PLANNING

Are the symptoms controlled?
Patient's symptoms should normally be well controlled before they are discharged from an in-patient unit.

Is the patient's condition stable?
A patient's condition should normally be stable before discharge is considered. If their conditions is deteriorating every few days its suggest that the terminal phase is near, some dying patients want to return home to die. This involves an open discussion with the patient and relatives that this is the intended plan.

Does the patient want to go home?
If a patient wants to go home the decisions depend mainly on whether the patient is self caring and how much support is available at home. If the patient insists on going home without any good support then a trial period at home with the option of re-admission may be the solution.

	Self-Caring	Not Self-Caring
Patient wants to go home	Home plus follow-up	Rehabilitation(?) Support relatives, Care package Trial at home(?)
Patient does not want to go home	Emotional and Psychological Support	Nursing Home (+/- Health Care funding)

Is the patient eligible for Health Care funding?
The key requirements are complex needs (needing specialist palliative care monitoring) and a progressive illness. (Note the same patient can be "stable" in hospice terms and yet have a "deteriorating condition" in terms of Health Care funding.)

Have patient's needs been assessed?
Patient's are entitled in law to a full needs-led assessment by a social worker (inpatient) or care manager (outpatient). Patient's not eligible for Health Care funding may still be placed in a Nursing Home if they have "very high needs for services" e.g. dependent day and night or needing constant supervision, or help with all household affairs, or if the home environment is hazardous, or with poor social support.

Are the plans realistic?
Lack of local funding or local services may restrict what is possible. If a highly dependent patient wants to be cared for at home it is not always possible. This may need to be explained to the patient

Have relevant communications happened?
The key to successful discharge home is often face to face contact between the in-patient team and the District Nurses.

DYING

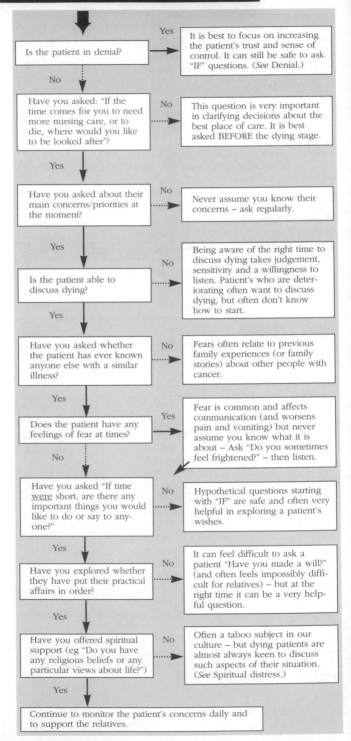

Is the patient in denial? — Yes → It is best to focus on increasing the patient's trust and sense of control. It can still be safe to ask "IF" questions. (*See* Denial.)

No

Have you asked: "If the time comes for you to need more nursing care, or to die, where would you like to be looked after"? — No → This question is very important in clarifying decisions about the best place of care. It is best asked BEFORE the dying stage.

Yes

Have you asked about their main concerns/priorities at the moment? — No → Never assume you know their concerns – ask regularly.

Yes

Is the patient able to discuss dying? — No → Being aware of the right time to discuss dying takes judgement, sensitivity and a willingness to listen. Patient's who are deteriorating often want to discuss dying, but often don't know how to start.

Yes

Have you asked whether the patient has ever known anyone else with a similar illness? — No → Fears often relate to previous family experiences (or family stories) about other people with cancer.

Yes

Does the patient have any feelings of fear at times? — Yes → Fear is common and affects communication (and worsens pain and vomiting) but never assume you know what it is about – Ask "Do you sometimes feel frightened?" – then listen.

No

Have you asked "If time were short, are there any important things you would like to do or say to anyone?" — No → Hypothetical questions starting with "IF" are safe and often very helpful in exploring a patient's wishes.

Yes

Have you explored whether they have put their practical affairs in order? — No → It can feel difficult to ask a patient "Have you made a will?" (and often feels impossibly difficult for relatives) – but at the right time it can be a very helpful question.

Yes

Have you offered spiritual support (eg "Do you have any religious beliefs or any particular views about life?") — No → Often a taboo subject in our culture – but dying patients are almost always keen to discuss such aspects of their situation. (*See* Spiritual distress.)

Yes

Continue to monitor the patient's concerns daily and to support the relatives.

What do dying patients need?

People facing death are as individual as people living life, and their specific needs vary. However after the initial crisis of knowledge, and the change it brings (internal and external) there is generally a period of emotional adjustment to the potential losses and fears.

When should a patient adjust to dying?

Adjustment to dying is a question of balance. Every patient has the right to be aware when time is short so they can put their affairs in order (if they want to). On the other hand if a patient adjusts to dying too soon they can experience a "social death" before their physical death, and end up with a long frustrating period of "waiting to die" with no meaningful connection to their previous life.

---

3 PHASES OF DYING

CRISIS (denial, anger, bargaining, searching)
→ **ADJUSTMENT** (facing fears, grieving for losses)
→ **ACCEPTANCE** (new "role", "letting go")

Has the patient expressed their grief for their losses?

Dying involves adjusting to a whole series of losses and disappointment, and each one causes grief. Often the earlier losses (mobility, independence, driving, social roles, physical appearance, feeling secure about life, a family future etc. etc.) are much harder to cope with than dying itself. Patients are more likely to cope effectively with a loss if they have had an opportunity to express their grief for previous losses.

Are the patient's fears realistic?

Dying patients often have fears, but professionals need to ask about them (not assume they know what they are). Common fears include separation (from loved ones, pets, home), becoming a burden, losing control, pain, making a mess, dying, being dead or leaving responsibilities unmet. Less obvious fears include fear of seeing fear in others and fear of feeling even more frightened as death approaches. Many fears are unrealistic and based on the false assumption that dying will bring a peak of suffering. Open, clear discussion of what dying will probably involve (for the patient and family) and what professionals can do to help can greatly reduce fears.

How do I respond to questions about prognosis?

A good response to the questions "How long have I got?" is often: "How long are you hoping for?" Some patients want as long as possible, others feel so exhausted that they are genuinely relieved to know they will die soon. Knowing what the patient is hoping for helps you to respond appropriately to their concerns:

   e.g. – "You may have a lot longer than you think"
   OR – "Time is short for you now".

See also: Terminal Phase (which focuses more on the physical issues).

DYSPHAGIA

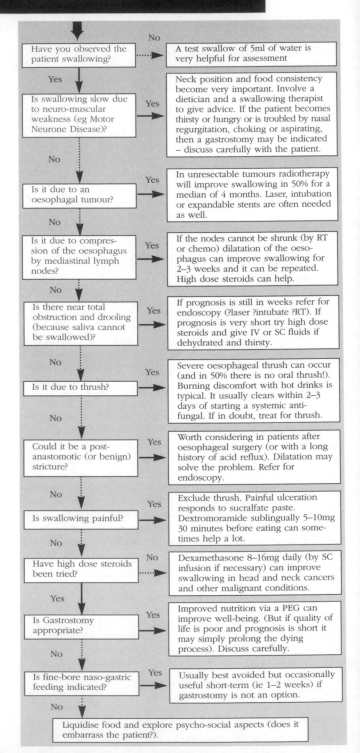

Have you observed the patient swallowing? — No → A test swallow of 5ml of water is very helpful for assessment

Yes ↓

Is swallowing slow due to neuro-muscular weakness (eg Motor Neurone Disease)? — Yes → Neck position and food consistency become very important. Involve a dietician and a swallowing therapist to give advice. If the patient becomes thirsty or hungry or is troubled by nasal regurgitation, choking or aspirating, then a gastrostomy may be indicated – discuss carefully with the patient.

No ↓

Is it due to an oesophagal tumour? — Yes → In unresectable tumours radiotherapy will improve swallowing in 50% for a median of 4 months. Laser, intubation or expandable stents are often needed as well.

No ↓

Is it due to compression of the oesophagus by mediastinal lymph nodes? — Yes → If the nodes cannot be shrunk (by RT or chemo) dilatation of the oesophagus can improve swallowing for 2–3 weeks and it can be repeated. High dose steroids can help.

No ↓

Is there near total obstruction and drooling (because saliva cannot be swallowed)? — Yes → If prognosis is still in weeks refer for endoscopy (?laser ?intubate ?RT). If prognosis is very short try high dose steroids and give IV or SC fluids if dehydrated and thirsty.

No ↓

Is it due to thrush? — Yes → Severe oesophageal thrush can occur (and in 50% there is no oral thrush!). Burning discomfort with hot drinks is typical. It usually clears within 2–3 days of starting a systemic anti-fungal. If in doubt, treat for thrush.

No ↓

Could it be a post-anastomotic (or benign) stricture? — Yes → Worth considering in patients after oesophageal surgery (or with a long history of acid reflux). Dilatation may solve the problem. Refer for endoscopy.

No ↓

Is swallowing painful? — Yes → Exclude thrush. Painful ulceration responds to sucralfate paste. Dextromoramide sublingually 5–10mg 30 minutes before eating can sometimes help a lot.

No ↓

Have high dose steroids been tried? — No → Dexamethasone 8–16mg daily (by SC infusion if necessary) can improve swallowing in head and neck cancers and other malignant conditions.

Yes ↓

Is Gastrostomy appropriate? — Yes → Improved nutrition via a PEG can improve well-being. (But if quality of life is poor and prognosis is short it may simply prolong the dying process). Discuss carefully.

No ↓

Is fine-bore naso-gastric feeding indicated? — Yes → Usually best avoided but occasionally useful short-term (ie 1–2 weeks) if gastrostomy is not an option.

No ↓

Liquidise food and explore psycho-social aspects (does it embarrass the patient?).

What is the main problem?
Is the problem reduced hydration, reduced nutrition, loss of social pleasure, pain on swallowing or risk of aspiration?. Are the relatives distressed by the poor food intake?

What is the cause?
Patients localise the level accurately in 99% of cases. Observe a TEST SWALLOW of 5ml of water to visualize the problem. Is it a problem with saliva, chewing (dentures or teeth), oral cavity (mucosal pain, poor closure) tongue movement ("ta" tests anterior tongue, "ka" tests posterior tongue) elevation of palate (nasal regurgitation) or closure of epiglottis (coughing, choking) elevation of larynx or oesophageal peristalsis?. Note that the gag reflex is irrelevant to the swallowing reflex.

Is it a delayed pharyngeal phase?
Pharyngeal function can be assessed at the bedside. Laryngeal elevation is easy to feel and normally takes 1 second. If it takes 5 seconds or longer swallowing becomes hard work and there is a risk of inadequate intake. Changing neck and body position (and food consistency) can still improve swallowing – involve a swallowing therapist and dietician. If it takes longer than 10 seconds then non-oral feeding will usually be needed. Is it worsened by drugs (eg metoclopramide)?

Is aspiration occurring?
After a test swallow ask the patient to say "Ahh". A gurgling noise means aspiration is probably occurring. Aspiration is symptomless in 40% of cases. In 60% it causes choking, coughing, drooling or recurrent chest infections. Consider changing the neck position (holding neck forward reduces it) and food changing consistency may help (eg semi-solids like yoghurt and custard can reduce aspiration occurring). If severe, non-oral feeding is necessary. Barium swallow is unhelpful (and can be dangerous). Video fluoroscopy will demonstrate the cause of problem and show how much aspiration is occurring.

Is non-oral feeding needed?
- fine-bore NG tube (1-2 week only)
- PEG
- open gastrostomy (eg oesophageal block)
- pharyngostomy (for oral tumours)

Improved nutrition can help well-being (and relieve nutritional deficiencies) and should be considered early in patients with a reasonable prognosis. Seek advice of specialist nutritional nurse. (Note that it is easier to start non-oral feeding than to stop.)

Is the patient in the last few days?
The key decision is: "Is the patient thirsty?" If not, focus on mouth care. (see Dehydration).

See also: Nutrition

DYSPNOEA

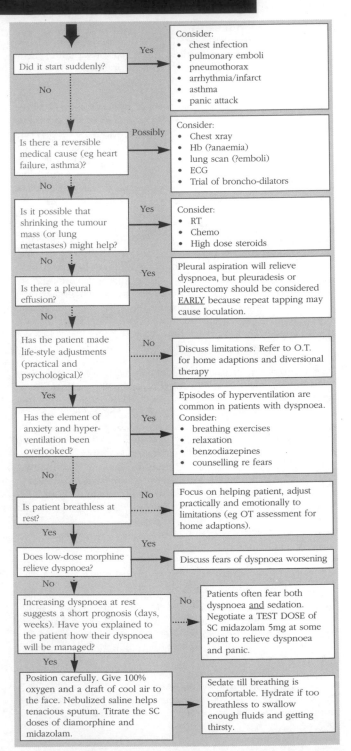

Did it start suddenly? — **Yes** →

Consider:
- chest infection
- pulmonary emboli
- pneumothorax
- arrhythmia/infarct
- asthma
- panic attack

No ↓

Is there a reversible medical cause (eg heart failure, asthma)? — **Possibly** →

Consider:
- Chest xray
- Hb (?anaemia)
- lung scan (?emboli)
- ECG
- Trial of broncho-dilators

No ↓

Is it possible that shrinking the tumour mass (or lung metastases) might help? — **Yes** →

Consider:
- RT
- Chemo
- High dose steroids

No ↓

Is there a pleural effusion? — **Yes** →

Pleural aspiration will relieve dyspnoea, but pleuradesis or pleurectomy should be considered <u>EARLY</u> because repeat tapping may cause loculation.

No ↓

Has the patient made life-style adjustments (practical and psychological)? — **No** →

Discuss limitations. Refer to O.T. for home adaptions and diversional therapy

Yes ↓

Has the element of anxiety and hyper-ventilation been overlooked? — **Yes** →

Episodes of hyperventilation are common in patients with dyspnoea. Consider:
- breathing exercises
- relaxation
- benzodiazepines
- counselling re fears

No ↓

Is patient breathless at rest? — **No** →

Focus on helping patient, adjust practically and emotionally to limitations (eg OT assessment for home adaptions).

Yes ↓

Does low-dose morphine relieve dyspnoea? — **Yes** →

Discuss fears of dyspnoea worsening

No ↓

Increasing dyspnoea at rest suggests a short prognosis (days, weeks). Have you explained to the patient how their dyspnoea will be managed? — **No** →

Patients often fear both dyspnoea <u>and</u> sedation. Negotiate a TEST DOSE of SC midazolam 5mg at some point to relieve dyspnoea and panic.

Yes ↓

Position carefully. Give 100% oxygen and a draft of cool air to the face. Nebulized saline helps tenacious sputum. Titrate the SC doses of diamorphine and midazolam. →

Sedate till breathing is comfortable. Hydrate if too breathless to swallow enough fluids and getting thirsty.

Did the dyspnoea (breathlessness) start suddenly?

Sudden onset over hours suggests a medical cause (myocardial infarct, embolus, arrythmia, asthma). These may need excluding before diagnosing a first panic attack. Consider a CXR and ECG. Worsening over days suggests a chest infection or pleural effusion. Worsening over weeks suggests anaemia or tumour progression.

Is it mainly on exertion?

Breathlessness on exertion is the commonest problem (which may gradually worsen). The focus of management is on non-drug measures. The patient has to learn to *avoid* distressing breathlessness by adjusting their life-style (a home visit by an occupational therapist can be very helpful) and has to learn to *cope* with the sensation when it occurs without panicking (breathing exercises and relaxation techniques taught by a physiotherapist can be very effective).

What does it prevent the patient from doing?

This is a useful question to assess the impact on quality of life. Most patients have difficulty coping with some aspects of change in life-style, and need help adjusting (practical and emotional).

Should breathless patients still take exercise?

Suprisingly breathless patients should still exercise to the limits of comfort, because exercise has a positive effect physically and mentally. Relatives are often over-protective and try to stop the patient from doing anything. An assessment of exercise tolerance by the doctor, using a simple walking test, can give the patient and relatives more confidence.

Is the patient breathless at rest?

Difficulty breathing even at rest (or taking a long time to recover from exertion) is when low dose morphine is considered (a starting dose is 2.5mg morphine 4 hourly) and it can greatly reduce the distressing sensation of breathlessness.

Is the patient getting episodes of hyperventilation?

Breathlessness is frightening and many patients with breathlessness *also* get episodes of hyperventilation, and sometimes panic. A helpful point is that breathing tends to ease slightly with exertion if hyperventilation is the main problem. Ask if the patient feels frightened at times. Most patients fear it will worsen and they will die gasping for breath. Open discussion of fears (usually about it worsening) and how it can be controlled (if it worsens) can help a lot.

How is severe breathlessness at rest managed?

This can occur in the last few days of life, and breathing can become more and more distressing. SC infusion of diamorphine plus midazolam in carefully titrated doses is effective. Continuous oxygen is also helpful (but constant fears about the oxygen cylinders running out is not, so change them regularly). Skilled nursing, and careful positioning and moving of the patient make all the difference. Make sure the environment feels safe and calm and that the patient is not left alone. Patients often fear it getting worse, but also fear sedation in case they stop breathing altogether. Negotiate the idea of a TEST DOSE OF MIDAZOLAM 5mg IM with the patient. This gives sedation and relief without depressing respiration, and wears off after an hour or so. If the patient is too breathless to speak arrange a signal so they can ask to try it when they feel ready, which gives them an important sense of control.

EMERGENCIES

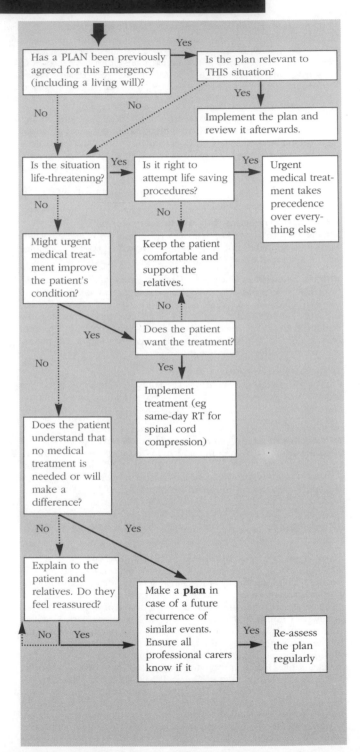

Has a PLAN been previously agreed for this Emergency (including a living will)? → **Yes** → Is the plan relevant to THIS situation?

→ **Yes** → Implement the plan and review it afterwards.

No

No

Is the situation life-threatening? → **Yes** → Is it right to attempt life saving procedures? → **Yes** → Urgent medical treatment takes precedence over everything else

No

No

Might urgent medical treatment improve the patient's condition? → Keep the patient comfortable and support the relatives.

Yes

No

Does the patient want the treatment? → **No**

Yes → Implement treatment (eg same-day RT for spinal cord compression)

Does the patient understand that no medical treatment is needed or will make a difference?

No   **Yes**

Explain to the patient and relatives. Do they feel reassured? → **No** / **Yes** → Make a **plan** in case of a future recurrence of similar events. Ensure all professional carers know if it → **Yes** → Re-assess the plan regularly

Is this a <u>medical</u> emergency or a <u>social</u> emergency?
This flow chart is about <u>medical</u> emergencies. Sometimes "medical" emergencies are in reality social crises – be clear about the difference. Where do responsibilities lie?

Is immediate treatment needed?
Will rapid treatment have a better effect than delayed treatment? Common examples include spinal cord compression, relief of obstructive renal failure (with a stent or nephrostomy) treatment of hypercalcaemia with IV bisphosphates, fractures, allergic reactions, fits, severe pains, bleeding, urinary retention, stridor, severe anxiety or panic attacks, hyperventilation, psychotic episodes or terminal agitation.

Can emergencies be avoided?
An emergency can be defined as any situation for which there is no prearranged plan. Planning can reduce the likelihood of emergencies, eg if a patient has a tracheotomy that is beginning to fail the question needs to be discussed <u>now</u>; "What will happen if it blocks (in the night) - what will we do?". This will also need to be discussed with the patient and usually the relatives.

Is the "emergency" due to progression of the underlying disease?
The problem for patients (and relatives) is that they are often unsure (and frightened) whenever a change occurs *in case* it's an emergency - ie in case urgent treatment would be significantly better than delayed treatment. In a progressive condition such frightening moments tend to occur around the time of a deterioration in condition, which can be step-wise:

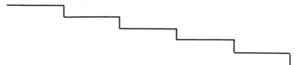

Careful explanation is often enough to diffuse such "emergencies" which are due to fear.

Have you made a plan?
Plans should be <u>transportable</u> and should apply wherever the patient is being cared for (home, hospital, hospice).

<u>See also</u>: Deterioration

ETHICAL PROBLEMS

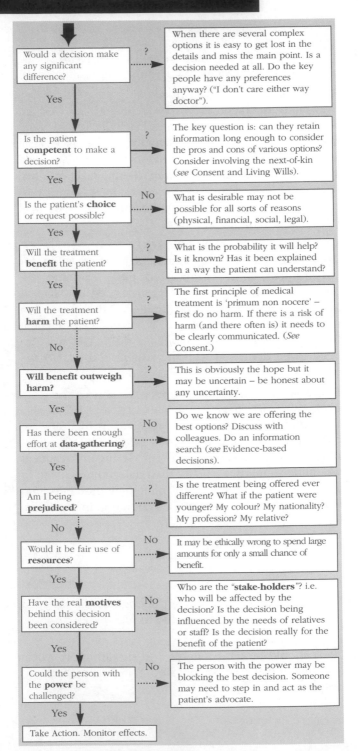

| Would a decision make any significant difference? | ? | When there are several complex options it is easy to get lost in the details and miss the main point. Is a decision needed at all. Do the key people have any preferences anyway? ("I don't care either way doctor"). |

Yes

| Is the patient **competent** to make a decision? | ? | The key question is: can they retain information long enough to consider the pros and cons of various options? Consider involving the next-of-kin (*see* Consent and Living Wills). |

Yes

| Is the patient's **choice** or request possible? | No | What is desirable may not be possible for all sorts of reasons (physical, financial, social, legal). |

Yes

| Will the treatment **benefit** the patient? | ? | What is the probability it will help? Is it known? Has it been explained in a way the patient can understand? |

Yes

| Will the treatment **harm** the patient? | ? | The first principle of medical treatment is 'primum non nocere' – first do no harm. If there is a risk of harm (and there often is) it needs to be clearly communicated. (*See* Consent.) |

No

| **Will benefit outweigh harm?** | ? | This is obviously the hope but it may be uncertain – be honest about any uncertainty. |

Yes

| Has there been enough effort at **data-gathering**? | No | Do we know we are offering the best options? Discuss with colleagues. Do an information search (*see* Evidence-based decisions). |

Yes

| Am I being **prejudiced**? | ? | Is the treatment being offered ever different? What if the patient were younger? My colour? My nationality? My profession? My relative? |

No

| Would it be fair use of **resources**? | No | It may be ethically wrong to spend large amounts for only a small chance of benefit. |

Yes

| Have the real **motives** behind this decision been considered? | No | Who are the "**stake-holders**"? i.e. who will be affected by the decision? Is the decision being influenced by the needs of relatives or staff? Is the decision really for the benefit of the patient? |

Yes

| Could the person with the **power** be challenged? | No | The person with the power may be blocking the best decision. Someone may need to step in and act as the patient's advocate. |

Yes

Take Action. Monitor effects.

What is the best option?

The central problem is this: there is no set of ethical principles or decision-making principles that can guarantee a correct decision (the main aim being for benefit to outweigh harm). Therefore the decision-making process needs to be as good as possible.

Could the treatment harm the patients?

There is often a risk of harmful side-effects. The problem is how far to explain all the potential risks for the patient (eg some drugs have a very long list of possible side-effects – should we inform the patient of them all?). Another problem is the question of balance. Take chemotherapy treatment as an example. We often know for sure it will cause harmful side-effects so the action "first do no harm" does not really apply – it is a question of considering the balance of side-effects to the advantages of treatment (the pros and cons), which will always be a matter of judgement.

Will others be affected by the decision?

The decision may impact on others. For example a patient may decide they want to be nursed at home, but the carers may feel they are unable to cope at the moment. Relevant others may need to be included in the discussion and the decision-making process.

What about patient choice?

The recent focus on patient autonomy has helped to re-empower patients (who have traditionally been very vulnerable) but the truth is that none of us are completely autonomous ("no man is an island"). At first glance it may seem that difficult decisions simply come down to the patient's choice but patients, like the rest of us, are not free to make choices that are illegal or that will harm others. The patient's rights and responsibilities have to be seen in the context of the rights and responsibilities of those around them (including the professional staff). In reality the patient, like the rest of us, has limited choices.

See also: Consent, Decision-making IV

EVIDENCE-BASED DECISIONS

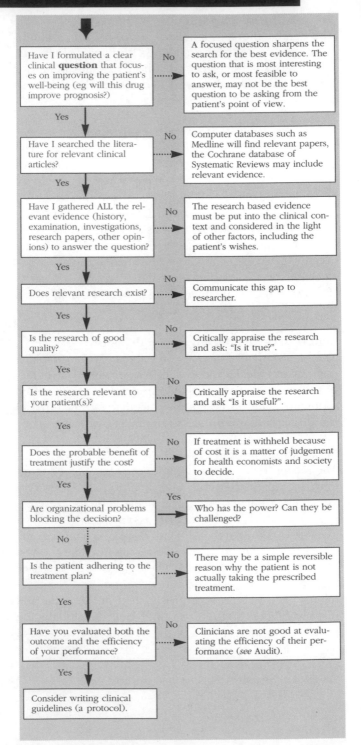

Have I formulated a clear clinical **question** that focuses on improving the patient's well-being (eg will this drug improve prognosis?)

No → A focused question sharpens the search for the best evidence. The question that is most interesting to ask, or most feasible to answer, may not be the best question to be asking from the patient's point of view.

Yes ↓

Have I searched the literature for relevant clinical articles?

No → Computer databases such as Medline will find relevant papers, the Cochrane database of Systematic Reviews may include relevant evidence.

Yes ↓

Have I gathered ALL the relevant evidence (history, examination, investigations, research papers, other opinions) to answer the question?

No → The research based evidence must be put into the clinical context and considered in the light of other factors, including the patient's wishes.

Yes ↓

Does relevant research exist?

No → Communicate this gap to researcher.

Yes ↓

Is the research of good quality?

No → Critically appraise the research and ask: "Is it true?".

Yes ↓

Is the research relevant to your patient(s)?

No → Critically appraise the research and ask "Is it useful?".

Yes ↓

Does the probable benefit of treatment justify the cost?

No → If treatment is withheld because of cost it is a matter of judgement for health economists and society to decide.

Yes ↓

Are organizational problems blocking the decision?

Yes → Who has the power? Can they be challenged?

No ↓

Is the patient adhering to the treatment plan?

No → There may be a simple reversible reason why the patient is not actually taking the prescribed treatment.

Yes ↓

Have you evaluated both the outcome and the efficiency of your performance?

No → Clinicians are not good at evaluating the efficiency of their performance (*see* Audit).

Yes ↓

Consider writing clinical guidelines (a protocol).

EVIDENCE-BASED DECISIONS

What is Evidence-based medicine?

"Evidence-based medicine is the conscientious, explicit and judicious use of current best evidence in making decisions about the care of individual patients and means integrating individual clinical expertise with the best available external clinical evidence from systematic research"

(Sacket, et al 1996)

How good is the evidence?

The strength of the evidence is obviously relevant when making clinical decisions. Ask yourself "How strong is the evidence I am using?"

STRENGTH OF EVIDENCE

- Review of RCT's
- RCT (Randomised controlled trial)
- Non-randomised trial
- Multi-centre experience
- Respected opinion
- "Someone told me"

Is the evidence relevant to this patient?

Most of the time we do not have firm research-based evidence for best clinical practice and we are trying to make optimum judgements in the face of uncertainty. Even when the evidence is clear and definite it still needs to be integrated into the unique situation of the individual patient.

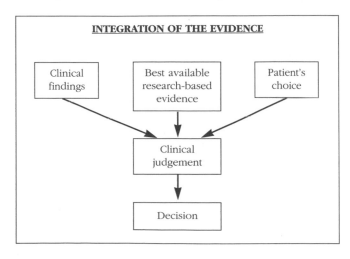

INTEGRATION OF THE EVIDENCE

Clinical findings → Clinical judgement

Best available research-based evidence → Clinical judgement

Patient's choice → Clinical judgement

Clinical judgement → Decision

EXPLANATION

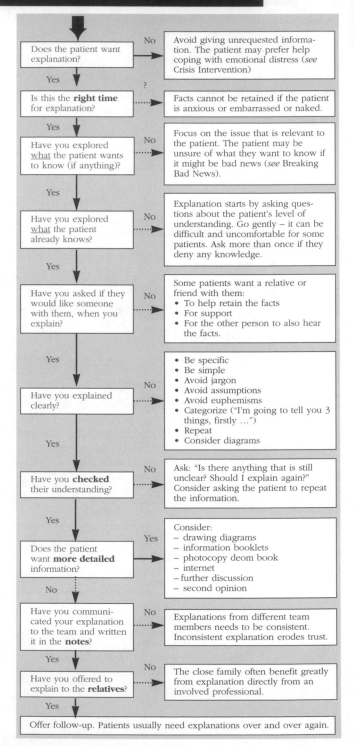

Does the patient want explanation?	No →	Avoid giving unrequested information. The patient may prefer help coping with emotional distress (*see* Crisis Intervention)
↓ Yes		
Is this the **right time** for explanation?	? ⋯⋯►	Facts cannot be retained if the patient is anxious or embarrassed or naked.
↓ Yes		
Have you explored <u>what</u> the patient wants to know (if anything)?	No ⋯⋯►	Focus on the issue that is relevant to the patient. The patient may be unsure of what they want to know if it might be bad news (*see* Breaking Bad News).
↓ Yes		
Have you explored <u>what</u> the patient already knows?	No ⋯⋯►	Explanation starts by asking questions about the patient's level of understanding. Go gently – it can be difficult and uncomfortable for some patients. Ask more than once if they deny any knowledge.
↓ Yes		
Have you asked if they would like someone with them, when you explain?	No ⋯⋯►	Some patients want a relative or friend with them: • To help retain the facts • For support • For the other person to also hear the facts.
↓ Yes		
Have you explained clearly?	No ⋯⋯►	• Be specific • Be simple • Avoid jargon • Avoid assumptions • Avoid euphemisms • Categorize ("I'm going to tell you 3 things, firstly …") • Repeat • Consider diagrams
↓ Yes		
Have you **checked** their understanding?	No ⋯⋯►	Ask: "Is there anything that is still unclear? Should I explain again?" Consider asking the patient to repeat the information.
↓ Yes		
Does the patient want **more detailed** information?	Yes ⋯⋯►	Consider: – drawing diagrams – information booklets – photocopy deom book – internet – further discussion – second opinion
↓ No		
Have you communicated your explanation to the team and written it in the **notes**?	No ⋯⋯►	Explanations from different team members needs to be consistent. Inconsistent explanation erodes trust.
↓ Yes		
Have you offered to explain to the **relatives**?	No ⋯⋯►	The close family often benefit greatly from explanation directly from an involved professional.
↓ Yes		

Offer follow-up. Patients usually need explanations over and over again.

What is explanation?

Explaining is fact-centered and professional-centred discussion. It is useful when describing medical procedures or treatments. It is the style of the technical expert, or teacher, which is useful for giving information or instruction.

What are the aims of explanation?

The aims of explanation are to convey information, clarify decisions, reduce uncertainty and increase trust. Any new symptom can be very frightening when you have cancer. Even explaining that various symptoms part of the same disease process can make the situation feel more manageable.

How does explanation differ from advice?

There are 4 different types of discussion with patients: explaining, advising, counselling and manipulating. We may use several types in a single conversation. They differ according to whether the main focus is on facts or feelings, and whether the discussion is centred on the patient or the professional. Explanation is less appropriate when discussing management options (when advising is more appropriate) or when discussing feelings (counselling). Avoid manipulation.

TYPES OF CONSULTATION		
	PATIENT CENTRED	PROFESSIONAL CENTRED
FACT CENTRED	**Advice**	**EXPLANATION**
FEELINGS CENTRED	**Counselling**	**Manipulation**

Is the explanation consistent?

Medical care is increasingly delivered by multi-disciplinary teams. It is essential that explanation is consistent. If one professional says one thing, and another professional gives conflicting explanation, it erodes trust. There needs to be regular communication within the team about the explanation given to patients.

See also: Leadership

115

FAMILY CARE

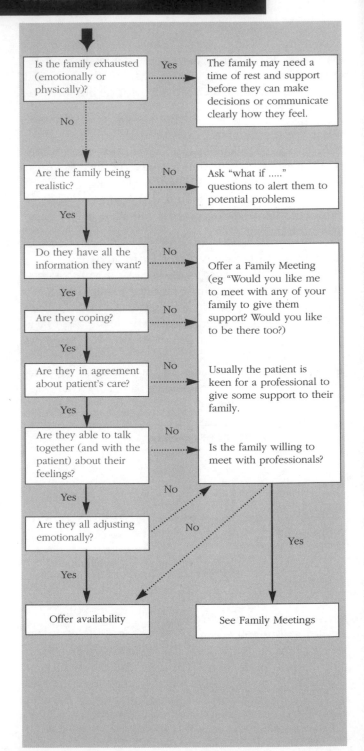

Is the family exhausted (emotionally or physically)? → **Yes** → The family may need a time of rest and support before they can make decisions or communicate clearly how they feel.

No ↓

Are the family being realistic? → **No** → Ask "what if ....." questions to alert them to potential problems

Yes ↓

Do they have all the information they want? → **No** →

Yes ↓

Are they coping? → **No** →

Offer a Family Meeting (eg "Would you like me to meet with any of your family to give them support? Would you like to be there too?)

Yes ↓

Are they in agreement about patient's care? → **No** → Usually the patient is keen for a professional to give some support to their family.

Yes ↓

Are they able to talk together (and with the patient) about their feelings? → **No** → Is the family willing to meet with professionals?

Yes ↓

Are they all adjusting emotionally? → **No** →

No / **Yes**

Yes ↓

Offer availability

See Family Meetings

116

What is a family?

At first glance the question "what is a family" seems obvious. But families are not all "nuclear" (with 2 parents and some children), and come in many shapes and sizes – (single parent, divorced or separated, multi-generational step-families, fostered, communal, and many others). The characteristics of any family, though, are emotional inter-dependence, a shared history and a future together – in other words a life-cycle of development. A dying person is leaving behind a living family system that will continue living.

Who is part of the family?

This is where drawing the family tree is so helpful. Who does the patient consider to be family?. Close friends may be more "family" than distant relatives. Are some important family members being overlooked (eg grandparents). Always get the patient's permission before talking with family members.

Why is family care important?

There are 5 reasons:

1. Most patients welcome an interest in their family, which helps them feel understood as a unique individual, not just "a number".

2. Many patients are very concerned about how their family is coping, and supporting the family is a good way to support the patient.

3. An anxious family makes it more difficult to care for the patient. In a sense family members are also patients (and some will be simultaneously visiting their GPs for anxiety-related symptoms).

4. Communication difficulties cause a lot of distress. Families often find it difficult to know how to talk with a close relative who is dying, and greatly benefit from a little bit of guidance.

5. Family support around the time of a death is effective "preventive psychiatry" reducing later psychological morbidity and modelling (especially for children) how to deal with future major losses.

FAMILY MEETINGS

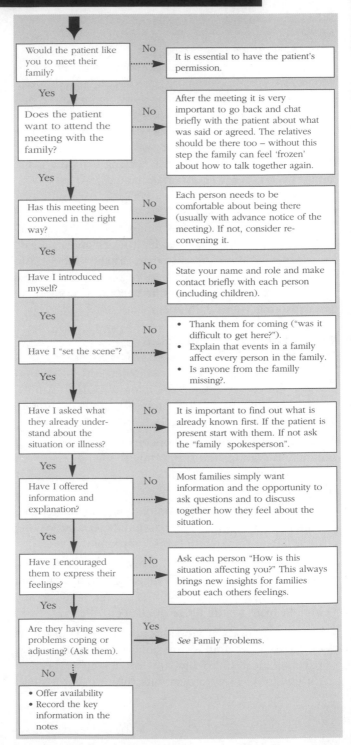

Would the patient like you to meet their family? — **No** → It is essential to have the patient's permission.

Yes

Does the patient want to attend the meeting with the family? — **No** → After the meeting it is very important to go back and chat briefly with the patient about what was said or agreed. The relatives should be there too – without this step the family can feel 'frozen' about how to talk together again.

Yes

Has this meeting been convened in the right way? — **No** → Each person needs to be comfortable about being there (usually with advance notice of the meeting). If not, consider re-convening it.

Yes

Have I introduced myself? — **No** → State your name and role and make contact briefly with each person (including children).

Yes

Have I "set the scene"? — **No** →
- Thank them for coming ("was it difficult to get here?").
- Explain that events in a family affect every person in the family.
- Is anyone from the family missing?.

Yes

Have I asked what they already understand about the situation or illness? — **No** → It is important to find out what is already known first. If the patient is present start with them. If not ask the "family spokesperson".

Yes

Have I offered information and explanation? — **No** → Most families simply want information and the opportunity to ask questions and to discuss together how they feel about the situation.

Yes

Have I encouraged them to express their feelings? — **No** → Ask each person "How is this situation affecting you?" This always brings new insights for families about each others feelings.

Yes

Are they having severe problems coping or adjusting? (Ask them). — **Yes** → *See* Family Problems.

No

- Offer availability
- Record the key information in the notes

How is the idea of family meetings introduced?
Ask the patient "would you like me to meet with your family I imagine they may be worrying about you. I will be happy to meet with them to explain about your illness. Would you also like to be there?".

How is the family meeting convened?
Convening a family meeting is a skill in itself. When and where should it be held? Who should invite the other family members? and How ?(e.g. face to face or by phone) Which professional(s) should attend? Timing is important (e.g. a lot of important family discussion can happen in the time before a family meeting takes place so it is sometimes a good idea to deliberately wait a few days.

Who should attend?
Who is considered to be part of the family network? Who does the patient want to be there? Is there anybody the patient does not want to be there? Drawing a family tree is very helpful at this point (See Family Tree).

How should the meeting start?
The professional is expected to start with discussion. Introduce yourself (and any colleagues). Thank the family for coming. Interact briefly with each person including children. Spend a short time socialising ("e.g. Did you have trouble getting here") mention how the meeting came about and discuss the aims of the meeting (usually to share information). At this point it can be helpful to ask a question and get the family talking (eg"What is the main concern for you as a family at the moment").

How should information be given?
Make sure you have all the facts (you may not need to explain much but it gives you confidence that you understand the situation medically). It is best to start by asking questions to find out the level of understanding of the family (eg "Could you help me first by explaining what you all understand about the situation and illness").

Should feelings be explored?
Family meetings are a very important opportunity to help the family to verbalise their feelings to each other. It can be very helpful to go round the circle and simply ask a question like " What is the most difficult part of this situation for each of you at the moment".

Should children attend?
Yes. Encourage the family to include children of all ages so they do not feel excluded. Talk at the youngest child's level. Very young children will need something quiet to occupy them such as drawing or crayoning (*See* Children).

FAMILY PROBLEMS

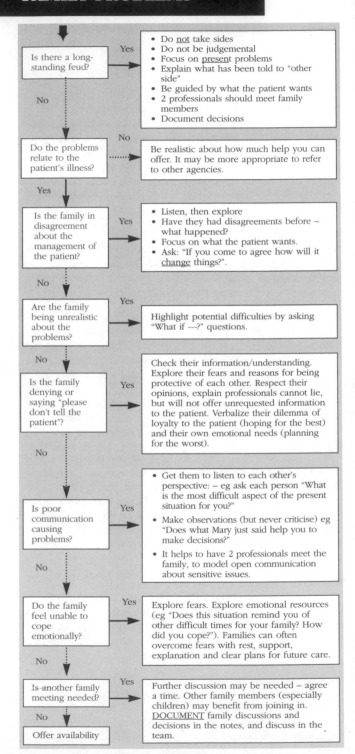

Is there a long-standing feud? — Yes →
- Do <u>not</u> take sides
- Do not be judgemental
- Focus on <u>present</u> problems
- Explain what has been told to "other side"
- Be guided by what the patient wants
- 2 professionals should meet family members
- Document decisions

No ↓

Do the problems relate to the patient's illness? — No ⋯→ Be realistic about how much help you can offer. It may be more appropriate to refer to other agencies.

Yes ↓

Is the family in disagreement about the management of the patient? — Yes →
- Listen, then explore
- Have they had disagreements before – what happened?
- Focus on what the patient wants.
- Ask: "If you come to agree how will it <u>change</u> things?".

No ↓

Are the family being unrealistic about the problems? — Yes → Highlight potential difficulties by asking "What if ---?" questions.

No ↓

Is the family denying or saying "please don't tell the patient"? — Yes → Check their information/understanding. Explore their fears and reasons for being protective of each other. Respect their opinions, explain professionals cannot lie, but will not offer unrequested information to the patient. Verbalize their dilemma of loyalty to the patient (hoping for the best) and their own emotional needs (planning for the worst).

No ↓

Is poor communication causing problems? — Yes →
- Get them to listen to each other's perspective: – eg ask each person "What is the most difficult aspect of the present situation for you?"
- Make observations (but never criticise) eg "Does what Mary just said help you to make decisions?"
- It helps to have 2 professionals meet the family, to model open communication about sensitive issues.

No ↓

Do the family feel unable to cope emotionally? — Yes → Explore fears. Explore emotional resources (eg "Does this situation remind you of other difficult times for your family? How did you cope?"). Families can often overcome fears with rest, support, explanation and clear plans for future care.

No ↓

Is another family meeting needed? — Yes → Further discussion may be needed – agree a time. Other family members (especially children) may benefit from joining in. <u>DOCUMENT</u> family discussions and decisions in the notes, and discuss in the team.

No ↓

Offer availability

Are the family problems long-lasting?

Be realistic about management aims. Communicate with other professions already involved (social worker, GP, probation officer etc). Dysfunctional families are trying to do their best. A death in the family can be an opportunity for them to see and do things differently, and to change the way they relate to each other, but if changing their behaviour is the aim, it is best if a professional with some family therapy training can be involved or consulted.

Are the patient's symptoms worse when the family visit?

This is due to anxiety and underlying fears – eg fear of how the family will cope in the future (especially if the patient is the "family mediator") or fear of not seeing them in the future (ie fear of dying) or fear that they may soon be discharged home and the family will not cope, or fear that the family do not understand how sick or bad they feel (hence exaggeration of the symptoms) etc. Usually it reflects parallel fears within the family. Work (gently) towards a family meeting to discuss their feelings honestly together.

Does the family seem "out of control" to the staff?

Problems can include children running out of control, adults who are drunk\abusive or feuding within the family. Hold a team meeting to discuss how to structure the attention they need. Set ground-rules for them and communicate them clearly to the family. Explain children must be supervised. Make it clear you will not tolerate disturbing behaviour and will call the police if necessary.

Are certain family members extremely distressed?

When one person in a family is particularly distressed it is tempting for staff to try to offer that individual a lot of time and support. However, it is usually much better in the palliative care setting to address the problem as part of the family pattern, and to try to offer help with and through the rest of the family as much as possible. Otherwise the person who is the "identified problem" can distract the team (and the family) away from the main issues.

Is it a very large family?

Staff (and patients) can feel overwhelmed by large families. Set a room aside for them when they are not at the bedside. Ask them to nominate a central spokesperson for staff to contact. Suggest they consider a rota so they can visit a few at a time. Ask the patient if he or she would like individual time with some of the family rather than always seeing them in groups (eg the patient may be getting little privacy with their partner).

FAMILY TREE

EXAMPLE OF A FAMILY TREE

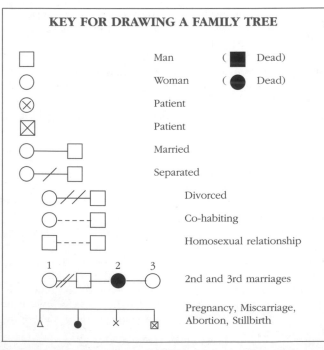

A family tree often highlights important decisions:

- Father, Harry, died of cancer (Does it "run in the family"?)
- Mother, Gwen, is frail ("Should we tell her?")
- Brother, John, lives abroad ("When should he come home?")
- Husband's first wife, Diane, died of cancer "in terrible pain" (explore what happened).
- First grandchild expected in four months. ("Will I live to see it born?")
- Son, Philip, is "never at home these days". (Is he too distressed to visit?)
- Step-daughter, Nancy, is estranged. (Should contact be re-established?)

KEY FOR DRAWING A FAMILY TREE

□	Man	(■ Dead)
○	Woman	(● Dead)
⊗	Patient	
⊠	Patient	
○—□	Married	
○—/—□	Separated	
○—//—□		Divorced
○----□		Co-habiting
□----□		Homosexual relationship
○ //□ ● ○ (1 2 3)		2nd and 3rd marriages
△ ● × ⊠		Pregnancy, Miscarriage, Abortion, Stillbirth

What is a family tree?

A Family Tree (genogram) is a diagramatic way of recording information about families. It usually covers 3 generations: Patients, parents and children. The initial diagram can be drawn by a doctor or nurse, but usually needs updating as the team learns more. It usually needs more than one session to get all the detailed information.

Is there a family tree in the notes?

A family tree is a very helpful and simple communication tool. At a glance you can see the structure of the family and the potential support available. It is also useful for remembering the names of important family members, and remembering to ask important questions (eg "has your new grandchild arrived yet?").

Do I have time to draw a family tree?

Drawing the diagram routinely take 5–10 minutes and provides helpful information on all patients. Time spent drawing a family tree is time invested, and it will certainly save time later. The concerns of the family are very relevant to managing the patient's problems. As time goes on it becomes increasingly helpful to know a bit about the family. Some of the issues raised by drawing a family tree may require more time (and it may then be more appropriate to arrange another session or to ask another team member to help.)

When do I introduce the idea?

Having listened to the patient's main concerns, and taken a full history (and just before examining the patient) is often a good moment to say "May I ask you a few questions about you and your family?" The few minutes spent discussing the family often transforms the consultation. The patient becomes aware of your wider perspective on their situation and often feels more relaxed and trustful.

What if the patient objects?

This happens rarely – most patients are delighted that you have an interest in their family. But occasionally a patient will say "Why do you need to know about my family?" It is helpful to explain that an illness usually affects everyone in a family (in different ways) and that it helps professionals to know about a patient's family support. If the patient is still defensive it is usually particularly important to find out why, and gently persisting with the idea of drawing a family tree (perhaps at a future consultation).

Note: When drawing a family tree keep each generation on the same line on the page. As their description of the family structure unfolds, it is sometimes necessary to re-start your drawing.

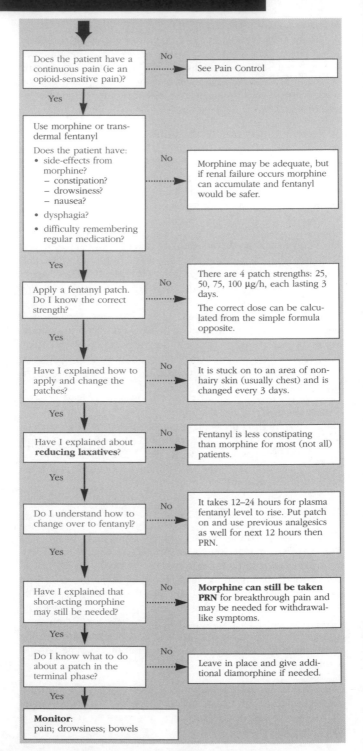

Does the patient have a continuous pain (ie an opioid-sensitive pain)?

No → See Pain Control

Yes

Use morphine or trans-dermal fentanyl

Does the patient have:
- side-effects from morphine?
  - constipation?
  - drowsiness?
  - nausea?
- dysphagia?
- difficulty remembering regular medication?

No → Morphine may be adequate, but if renal failure occurs morphine can accumulate and fentanyl would be safer.

Yes

Apply a fentanyl patch. Do I know the correct strength?

No → There are 4 patch strengths: 25, 50, 75, 100 µg/h, each lasting 3 days.

The correct dose can be calculated from the simple formula opposite.

Yes

Have I explained how to apply and change the patches?

No → It is stuck on to an area of non-hairy skin (usually chest) and is changed every 3 days.

Yes

Have I explained about **reducing laxatives**?

No → Fentanyl is less constipating than morphine for most (not all) patients.

Yes

Do I understand how to change over to fentanyl?

No → It takes 12–24 hours for plasma fentanyl level to rise. Put patch on and use previous analgesics as well for next 12 hours then PRN.

Yes

Have I explained that short-acting morphine may still be needed?

No → **Morphine can still be taken PRN** for breakthrough pain and may be needed for withdrawal-like symptoms.

Yes

Do I know what to do about a patch in the terminal phase?

No → Leave in place and give additional diamorphine if needed.

Yes

Monitor: pain; drowsiness; bowels

FENTANYL 1 – USAGE

Which patch strength is needed?

1. It is safe to start the 25mcg per hour patch if the patient has a constant pain which has not responded to moderate analgesics such as 60mg of Codeine 4 hourly or 2 Co-proxamol tablets 4 hourly. If the patient is already taking morphine and is being converted to a Fentanyl patch the correct patch strength can be calculated from the simple formula below.

4 hourly **oral** morphine (mg) (× 6 for 24h dose)	Fentanyl patch (mcg\hr)
5–20mg	25
30mg	50
45mg	75
60mg	100
120mg	200

When can the patch be started?

Apply the first patch at night together with the usual night dose of morphine then phase out the regular morphine dose the following day. The patient can still use immediate release morphine PRN for any breakthrough pain.

What are the side-effects?

Constipation, nausea or drowsiness can occur but there is a lower incidence than with morphine. Prolonged fever or a hot bath can increase fentanyl release and the chance of side-effects. Side-effects may persist for 24 hours after the patch is removed.

Is there a maximum dose?

There is no maximum dose of fentanyl but if the dose required exceeds 300mcg per hour (ie three 100 µg/h patches) consider additional or alternative analgesic therapy.

Is it a controlled drug?

Fentanyl is a controlled drug therefore prescriptions need to be written by the prescribing doctor in figures and words eg "Durogesic 25mgm per hour × 5 (five) patches, apply 1 patch every 3 days."

Can Fentanyl be used in the terminal phase?

Fentanyl should not be prescribed for the first time if the patient is in the terminal phase (ie their condition is deteriorating day by day) because it can be difficult to find the right dose quickly in a changing situation. However if the patient already has a Fentanyl patch this can be left in place and oral morphine or IM diamorphine can be given for breakthrough pain. A safe starting dose of IM diamorphine is 5mg per 25mcg per hour of Fentanyl.

What is the chance of a morphine withdrawal reaction?

About 10% of patients may experience transient withdrawal like symptoms when converted from morphine to fentanyl. The symptoms can last from a few days to 2 weeks and include diarrhoea, flu-like symptoms, yawning, runny nose, colic, anxiety, shivering and occasionally hallucinations. These symptoms respond within 30-60 minutes to a small dose of immediate release morphine eg Sevredol 10mg which can be given as often as necessary until it settles down.

See also: Fentanyl 2 – about the patch

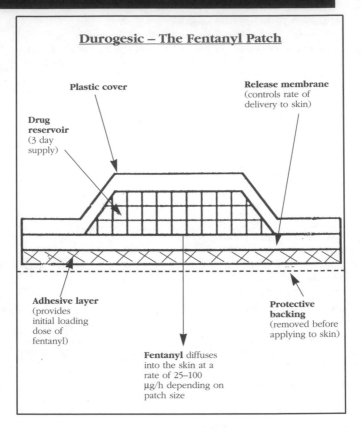

There are 4 patch strengths:

25 μg/hour
50 μg/hour
75 μg/hour
100 μg/hour

FENTANYL 2 – ABOUT THE PATCH

Where is the patch stuck on?
The patch is stuck on flat skin on the upper body (front or back) or upper arm. The skin should not have any cuts or spots and should not be hairy. Hairs can be cut with a pair of scissors but skin should not be shaved, as this may affect absorption. The skin should be dry. Soaps, oils or lotions should be avoided. The patch should be pressed firmly in place for 30 seconds and the edges of the patch pressed down.

How often is it changed?
The patch is normally changed every 3rd day (eg if it is put on at 9am on Wednesday it should be exchanged for a new patch at 9am of Saturday). Several days should elapse before a new patch is applied to the same area of skin.

Occasionally some patients notice that the analgesic effect falls after 60 hours, and it may then be necessary to change the patch every 2 days.

Can allergy to the patch occur?
Allergy is rare. Most skin reactions (redness or itching) resolve within 24 hours of removal of the patch. Occasionally they are troublesome and an alternative form of analgesia has to be found.

What if the patch falls off?
If a patch falls off it is safe to apply another replacement patch straight away and this new replacement patch will last a further 3 days. If the patch begins to peel off use Micropore or Tegaderm to hold it in place.

Is it waterproof?
The patch is waterproof for a shower, bath or swimming. The patch should not be worn under a tight elasticated band. Direct heat should be avoided as it can increase the rate of release of fentanyl (eg heat pads, hot water bottles, electric blankets, heat lamps, saunas, spa baths). Tell the patient to cover the patch with clothing if they sunbathe or use a sunbed.

What about used patches?
Used patches should be folded in half so that the sticky side sticks to itself and should be put back into its original pouch (which should therefore be kept when the patch is first opened). It is safe to discard the pouch in the household rubbish but keep out of the reach of children or pets.

GENETIC COUNSELLING

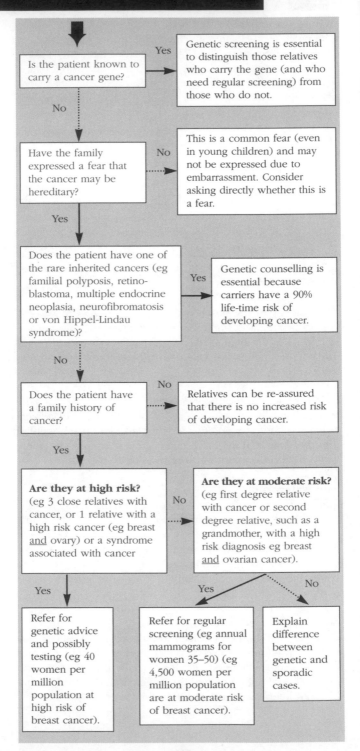

Is the patient known to carry a cancer gene?

Yes → Genetic screening is essential to distinguish those relatives who carry the gene (and who need regular screening) from those who do not.

No ↓

Have the family expressed a fear that the cancer may be hereditary?

No → This is a common fear (even in young children) and may not be expressed due to embarrassment. Consider asking directly whether this is a fear.

Yes ↓

Does the patient have one of the rare inherited cancers (eg familial polyposis, retino-blastoma, multiple endocrine neoplasia, neurofibromatosis or von Hippel-Lindau syndrome)?

Yes → Genetic counselling is essential because carriers have a 90% life-time risk of developing cancer.

No ↓

Does the patient have a family history of cancer?

No → Relatives can be re-assured that there is no increased risk of developing cancer.

Yes ↓

Are they at high risk? (eg 3 close relatives with cancer, or 1 relative with a high risk cancer (eg breast <u>and</u> ovary) or a syndrome associated with cancer

No → **Are they at moderate risk?** (eg first degree relative with cancer or second degree relative, such as a grandmother, with a high risk diagnosis eg breast <u>and</u> ovarian cancer).

Yes ↓

Refer for genetic advice and possibly testing (eg 40 women per million population at high risk of breast cancer).

Yes ↓

Refer for regular screening (eg annual mammograms for women 35–50) (eg 4,500 women per million population are at moderate risk of breast cancer).

No ↓

Explain difference between genetic and sporadic cases.

GENETIC COUNSELLING

Who needs Genetic Counselling?

Genetic testing is not necessary (as yet) for the majority of people. These notes offer guidelines for deciding which families to refer for genetic counselling or to the nearest cancer family-history clinic.

Can cancer run in families?

About 10% of patients with common cancers have a family history of relatives with cancer. Many of these will simply be coincidence (because cancer is a common condition) but some will reflect an inherited pre-disposition. The common familial cancers are:

FAMILIAL CANCER	GENE
Colon (non-polyposis)	hMSH2, hMLH1 hPMS1 and 2
Breast +/– ovary	BRCA 1
Breast/male breast	BRCA 2

These <u>familial cancers</u> are rare (about 1000 cases per year of each in the UK) but gene carriers have an 80% life-time risk of developing cancer, so genetic testing is important. 80% of families with dominant inheritance of breast cancer have one of these two genes. Individuals with a mutation in either of these genes have a 90% lifetime risk of developing breast cancer.

There are also some <u>inherited syndromes</u>, which carry about 80% life-time risk of developing cancer. They are rare (about 100 cases per year of each in the UK.)

Rare syndromes associated with cancer		
SYNDROME	**TUMOUR**	**GENE**
• Familial adenomatous polyposis	Colo-rectal	APC
• Retinoblastoma	Retina	RB1
• Multiple endocrine neoplasia – type 1	Pituitary Pancreas Parathyroid	MEN1
• Multiple endocrine neoplasia – type 2	Thyroid Adrenal	RET
• Neurofibromatosis – type 2	Acoustic neuroma Meningioma	NF2
• Von Hippel-Lindau	Phaeochromocytoma	VHL

What is "genetic testing"?

Genetic testing involves identifying the mutation in the faulty gene <u>then</u> offering genetic testing to unaffected individuals in the family. Even in families with a gene such as BRCA 1 there is a 50% chance of having inherited the good copy of the gene. It can take months to sequence a gene to look for a mutation, and present methods can only detect 80–90% of mutations.

GUIDELINES

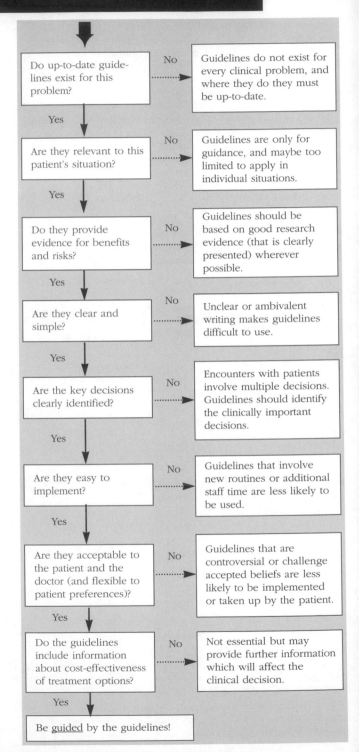

Do up-to-date guide-lines exist for this problem?

No → Guidelines do not exist for every clinical problem, and where they do they must be up-to-date.

Yes

Are they relevant to this patient's situation?

No → Guidelines are only for guidance, and maybe too limited to apply in individual situations.

Yes

Do they provide evidence for benefits and risks?

No → Guidelines should be based on good research evidence (that is clearly presented) wherever possible.

Yes

Are they clear and simple?

No → Unclear or ambivalent writing makes guidelines difficult to use.

Yes

Are the key decisions clearly identified?

No → Encounters with patients involve multiple decisions. Guidelines should identify the clinically important decisions.

Yes

Are they easy to implement?

No → Guidelines that involve new routines or additional staff time are less likely to be used.

Yes

Are they acceptable to the patient and the doctor (and flexible to patient preferences)?

No → Guidelines that are controversial or challenge accepted beliefs are less likely to be implemented or taken up by the patient.

Yes

Do the guidelines include information about cost-effectiveness of treatment options?

No → Not essential but may provide further information which will affect the clinical decision.

Yes

Be <u>guided</u> by the guidelines!

What are guidelines?

Guidelines (or protocols) are systematically developed statements intended to help doctors and patients to make better decisions about appropriate health care in specific circumstances. Simple guidelines can enable patients, doctors, purchasers and scientists to pool information more effectively. Authoritative guidelines involve a lot of consultation, so they are slow and expensive to produce.

When are guidelines useful?

Guidelines vary widely, but are often of poor quality, hard to update and often poorly used. Doctors are not good at following guidelines and protocols, compared to some other professionals. (For example airline pilots are excellent at following protocols – possibly because they die with their clients if things go wrong).

Guidelines are most likely to be used to change practise if they are locally developed, involve a specific educational strategy and have patient-specific reminders at the time of each consultation.

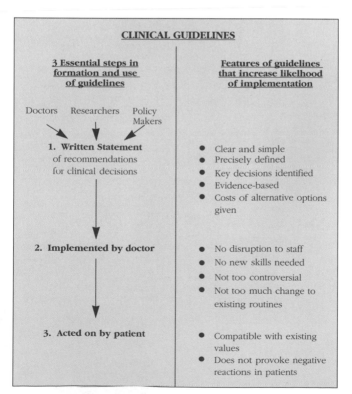

CLINICAL GUIDELINES

3 Essential steps in formation and use of guidelines	**Features of guidelines that increase likelihood of implementation**
Doctors Researchers Policy Makers	
1. Written Statement of recommendations for clinical decisions	• Clear and simple • Precisely defined • Key decisions identified • Evidence-based • Costs of alternative options given
2. Implemented by doctor	• No disruption to staff • No new skills needed • Not too controversial • Not too much change to existing routines
3. Acted on by patient	• Compatible with existing values • Does not provoke negative reactions in patients

HOME CARE

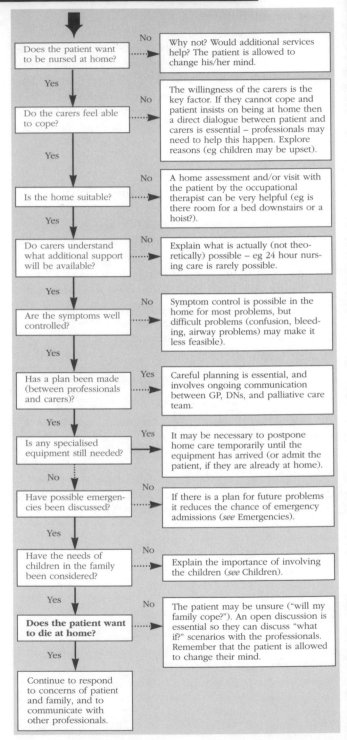

Does the patient want to be nursed at home?

→ No → Why not? Would additional services help? The patient is allowed to change his/her mind.

↓ Yes

Do the carers feel able to cope?

→ No → The willingness of the carers is the key factor. If they cannot cope and patient insists on being at home then a direct dialogue between patient and carers is essential – professionals may need to help this happen. Explore reasons (eg children may be upset).

↓ Yes

Is the home suitable?

→ No → A home assessment and/or visit with the patient by the occupational therapist can be very helpful (eg is there room for a bed downstairs or a hoist?).

↓ Yes

Do carers understand what additional support will be available?

→ No → Explain what is actually (not theoretically) possible – eg 24 hour nursing care is rarely possible.

↓ Yes

Are the symptoms well controlled?

→ No → Symptom control is possible in the home for most problems, but difficult problems (confusion, bleeding, airway problems) may make it less feasible).

↓ Yes

Has a plan been made (between professionals and carers)?

→ Yes → Careful planning is essential, and involves ongoing communication between GP, DNs, and palliative care team.

↓ Yes

Is any specialised equipment still needed?

→ Yes → It may be necessary to postpone home care temporarily until the equipment has arrived (or admit the patient, if they are already at home).

↓ No

Have possible emergencies been discussed?

→ No → If there is a plan for future problems it reduces the chance of emergency admissions (see Emergencies).

↓ Yes

Have the needs of children in the family been considered?

→ No → Explain the importance of involving the children (see Children).

↓ Yes

Does the patient want to die at home?

→ No → The patient may be unsure ("will my family cope?"). An open discussion is essential so they can discuss "what if?" scenarios with the professionals. Remember that the patient is allowed to change their mind.

↓ Yes

Continue to respond to concerns of patient and family, and to communicate with other professionals.

Is the home suitable?

Any home can be adapted to nurse a dying patient. More important than the surroundings are willing (and non-exhausted) carers and competent professionals. An OT assessment is often helpful.

Can the symptoms be managed in the home?

Most symptoms can be managed in the home. The particularly difficult problems are:

A	Airway problems
B	Bleeding (if heavy)
C	Confusion
D	Diarrhoea (if profuse)
E	Excruciating pain
F	Fits (if recurrent)

These symptoms may require admission to control them. Confusion in a patient erodes the carer's emotional strength for coping and is often the hardest symptom to cope with at home.

What emergency drugs are needed?

It is very useful if an "emergency box" of drugs can be kept in the patient's home, so that doctor's calling have drugs available if needed in the terminal phase. It should contain diamorphine, midazolam, hyosine, hydrobromide and metoclopramide for either IM injections or SC infusion and rectal diazepam (Sterolid) for emergency treatment of seizures.

What equipment is needed?

Useful equipment for a bed-bound patient includes special mattress, back-rest (eg Machett bag) bath seat, commode/urinal special cutlery (eg combined spoon and knife) non-slip mats (for food), beaker, flexible straws, electric fan, room-to-room intercom, angled table lamp, vacuum flask for hot/cold drinks, TV with remote, portable phone.

Useful <u>equipment for carers</u> includes liquidizer, microwave, ice-maker, handling straps or hoist, special mattress, drug card (to explain medication).

Useful <u>equipment for symptom control</u> may include syringe driver, deodoriser, nebulizer, TENS machine, compression pump for lymphoedema, portable suction, oxygen and incontinence sheath or pads.

Are the carers getting enough support?

This is often the key decision in maintaining the patient at home. If the carer's can't cope, the situation usually collapses and the patient ends up being admitted, often for something that could have easily been managed at home with a bit of professional guidance. Regular informal discussion with carers is essential.

INFORMATION

Is accurate information available?

We are increasingly being expected to base our decisions on the scientific evidence of controlled clinical trials, whenever possible. The section in this book on Evidence-based decisions describes how we should find and use the best available evidence for making decisions – in an ideal world.

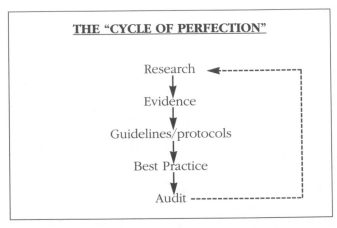

THE "CYCLE OF PERFECTION"

Research

↓

Evidence

↓

Guidelines/protocols

↓

Best Practice

↓

Audit

In reality it is still different. The chance of the relevant information being available when and where it is needed clinically is still very small. At the moment we often have to make clinical decisions without access to all the information that is actually available, (and we also have to make decisions about how much time to devote to chasing relevant information).

Is the information in a useful form?

A recent article called "Guidelines in general practice: the new Tower of Babel?" counted 855 different guidelines sent to GP's, 160 of them more than 10 pages long! The authors concluded: "this represents a large amount of information, but it is in an unmanageable form that does little to aid decision-making".

Simply disseminating information is not enough. In a recent article called "Where's the chief knowledge officer ?" Muir Gray concluded: "The truth is that the management of knowledge cannot be dealt with by individuals alone. The organisation in which individual clinicians work has to manage knowledge as well as it manages other resources".

See also: Evidence Based Decisions, Explanation, Guidelines.

How much information do patients need?

Doctors tend to under-estimate the amount of information patients want, An intelligent woman with cancer said "I needed to hear the information over and over again". Vicky Clement-Jones, a doctor who developed ovariarn cancer said "During my illness I was struck by the great need for information that both patients and their families had … they often needed explanation again and again" and she went on to found BACUP – an information service for cancer patients.

How do patients gain information?

In order to make decisions we need information. Patients gain information, (not always accurate), from a wide variety of sources.

SOME WAYS PATIENTS GAIN MEDICAL INFORMATION

- TV (soap operas, documentaries)
- GP\information leaflets
- Books\Library\Videos
- Magazines\Radio\Newspapers
- Medical experiences
- Family\friends
- Stories
- The Internet
- Other doctors

What sort of information helps?

Information is more likely to REACH the patient and meet the patient's needs if it meets the following criteria:

R Relevant to the patient
E Evidence-based
A Accessible
C Choice-enhancing
H Honestly presented (bias-free)

Is information ever unhelpful?

Information can be unhelpful, confusing and potentially dangerous if it is:

- Inaccurate
- Biased/dogmatic
- Incomprehensible
- Excessive ("analysis paralysis")

INTUITION

What is intuition?

In order to make decisions we need information. We gain the information we need in two different and distinct ways. There is rational (learned) information that is easy to talk about and discuss and there is intuition which is much more difficult to describe and talk about.

Intuition means knowledge based on feelings. We feel that we know something, but don't know how we know. No-one told us (as far as we can remember) Presumably intuitions involve an unconscious processing of verbal and non-verbal information.

Intuitions can be mistaken of course, but often (mysteriously) they are accurate. Women are said to make decisions based on intuition more than men.

Why is intuition important?

Accepting that some decision-making is intuitive is important because it encourages us to appreciate techniques like silence, waiting, pondering, day-dreaming, thinking aloud and an honest sharing of spontaneous thoughts in order to incorporate our unconscious mind into the process.

A case of intuition

A divorced man of 48 with advanced cancer of the colon told his doctor he wanted to ignore his illness as much as possible. He started dating a girl of 18 and took up several new interests including writing a novel. One day while dozing in his chair he had a "sort of nightmare" in which he "knew just two things" that he was not really Micheal Foster and he did not really live at 128 Sudborough Avenue. It frightened and disorientated him and he felt stunned by the force of the dream. After he had told the story he said quietly: "I don't know, I am not myself at the moment". After that day he began to adjust to the reality of his situation and to make more sensible decisions. He started seeing his grown up children again and began to sort out his financial affairs.

How do beliefs affect decisions?

Intuitions may relate to belifes. Sometimes a patient makes decisions that seem to make no sense to us, especially when the patient is from a different religious or ethnic group. The meaning and reasoning behind a patient's decision may only become clear by exploring their beliefs.

"I'M NOT TAKING YELLOW PILLS"

An intelligent academic patient with far-advanced cancer and massive leg oedema was prescribed some diuretics, but she kept "forgetting" to take them. When this behaviour was gently confronted she explained that she did not take them because they were yellow, and she had read that yellow colouring was bad for you, and could cause hyperactivity. This is an example of the influence of beliefs on medical decisions. It can be important to be aware of the opinions of the patient, however illogical they seem.

How can different beliefs be understood?

When a patient's decision seems illogical it can be helpful to explore the beliefs or attitudes which are affecting their decision. This involves being honest about your different perspective and asking questions that are more widely-focused than normal, eg "I'm sure you have good reasons for making that decision but it would help me to understand more if I knew more about how you are thinking. Do you know anyone else who has had this treatment?" etc. A useful idea from family therapy is that of "levels of context". Any conversation happens in the context of a lot of other influences.

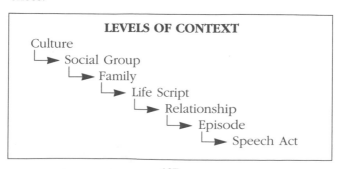

LEVELS OF CONTEXT

Culture
  → Social Group
    → Family
      → Life Script
        → Relationship
          → Episode
            → Speech Act

POSSIBLE RESULTS

	Disease present	**Disease absent**
Positive result	True positive (**sensitivity** of test)	False positive
Negative result	False negative	True negative (**specificity** of test)

Sensitivity is the ability of a test to correctly identify those people who have the disease in question. The greater the sensitivity, the fewer the false negatives.

$$\text{Sensitivity} = \frac{\text{True positive result}}{\text{True positive result + true negative result}} \times 100\%$$

A test is very **sensitive** if most positives are in fact positive (and only a small proportion are false positives). It is important to know how sensitive a test is.

Specificity is the ability of the test to correctly identify those individuals who do not have the disease in question. The greater the specificity, the fewer the false positives.

$$\text{Specificity} = \frac{\text{True negative result}}{\text{False positive result + true negative result}} \times 100\%$$

A test is very **specific** if most negatives are in fact negative (and only a small proportion are false negatives). It is important to know how specific the test is .

Predictive value is the ability of the test to identify those who truly have the disease amongst those who test positive for the disease.

$$\text{Predictive value} = \frac{\text{True positive result}}{\text{True positive result + false positive result}} \times 100\%$$

CASE HISTORY – A LOW HAEMOGLOBIN LEVEL

A patient with advanced breast cancer complaining of tiredness was found to have an Hb of 7.2g\dl and was admitted for a blood transfusion. Luckily the SHO re-checked the Hb level before commencing the blood transfusion and it was 12.5g\dl.

Will the test alter my management?

If an investigation will have no affect at all on management decisions (ie provide no useful information relevant to treatment, prognosis, or understanding the disease) it should not be performed. Instead, explain to the patient and relatives the reasoning behind the management, eg patient with far-advanced cancer often request scans "to see how it is progressing". Explain that clinical indicators (energy level, evidence of liver enlargement) are more appropriate measures of disease progression at this stage. Scan findings do not correlate (in any known way) with prognosis.

What are my real motives for requesting the test?

It can be tempting to request tests as a way of avoiding or postponing the discussion of distressing facts.

Could the result be a FALSE positive?

If a test has low sensitivity it means that there is a high chance of a *false positive*. Too many false positives will alarm too many patients unnecessarily and wastes resources on further tests. For example, an ESR can be elevated for lots of reasons, and would not be a good test for recurrence of, say, cancer of the prostate, whereas a PSA test would be sensitive. Choose the most sensitive test.

Could the result be a FALSE negative?

If the test has low specificity it means there is a high chance of a *false negative*. Too many false negatives means cases are being missed. For example, an Xray may not show an abnormality even though there is a bone metastasis present, and a bone scan may be more appropriate. Choose the most specific test.

When should test results be given to the patient?

As soon as possible – especially if the result significantly affects the patient's future (or if they feel it will) – because uncertainty is the hardest emotion of all to bear. If it is bad news consider how to tell them and find out if they want a relative or friend present (*see* Breaking Bad News).

Could the test result be wrong?

Diagnostic tests can enlarge our understanding of a disease but they can also erode our self-confidence about making independent judgements. We can become too dependent on investigations which are only an aid in decision-making (*see* Case History opposite).

JUDGEMENTS

"Good clinical medicine will always blend the art of uncertainty with the science of probability because clinical medicine consists of a few things we know, a few things we think we know (but probably don't) and lots of things we don't know at all"

CD Naylor

When making clinical decisions, "the facts must be taken into consideration but, on their own, do not tell the doctor what to do. The decision is a matter of judgement"

Bruce Charlton

What is Judgement?

Judgement can be defined as "making a decision or conclusion on the basis of indications and probabilities when the facts are not clearly known"

It is obvious that clinical decision-making relies on judgement. Facts, however accurate, are rarely enough. For example, even panels of experts discussing the appropriateness of a discrete procedures (eg colostomy) for particular cases will often disagree, (especially if they are from different counties). Even when a medical decision is black or white in the abstract, it often falls into a "grey zone" in the face of a patient's attitudes or individual needs.

We rarely have hard scientific data to guide our practice. In any clinical problem we usually have a number of options and the risk-benefit ratio of the various clinical options is often unknown. We often have to make clinical decisions in conditions of uncertainty. An important part of clinical decision-making is "nursing the uncertainty".

It is obvious that judgement comes into it, once we accept that medicine is 'not a science, but a rational science-using, interpretative activity undertaken for the care of the sick person' (Hudson Jones). Judgements may include how much the patient wants to be involved in making the decisions, and which issues have priority.

What factors can influence our judgements?

Cultural experience, social class, the beliefs of our own family, intellectual ability, life experience (eg the last patient), a patient's personality (eg openness), our attitude towards our professional role (eg helping vs autonomy), spiritual beliefs, current feelings and pressure of work can all influence our judgements.

Am I being prejudiced?

We all make decisions through "value glasses". What factors influence our choices?

EXPLORING PREJUDICES

Imagine a particular patient dying with a respiratory tract infection. Consider some of your management options. Decide what is appropriate:

- Wait?
- Sedate?
- Oral antibiotics?
- I.V. antibiotics?
- Physiotherapy?
- Combinations of the above?

Now see whether your decision is likely to alter with any of the following pieces of additional information?

- The patient is very unpopular
- The patient speaks no English
- Husband is a surgeon
- Children aged 3, 7, 10 and 12
- Parents visit tomorrow
- Sister is a physiotherapist
- Patient mentioned euthanasia to a nurse

How can I check out my own prejudice?

The internal influences on our decision-making are often invisible to us, which is why it is important to check difficult decisions with colleagues. Our internal judgements remain untested if they are not verbalized. Seeing how we agree or disagree with other people's views is the best way of understanding our own internal prejudices and "blind spots". This is discussed in more detail in the Introduction.

See Also: Probability.

STYLES OF DECISION-MAKING

Byrne and Long taped and analysed GP consultations
and found a variety of styles were needed, and used a
"power-shift" model to describe the varying involvement of the patient in decisions.

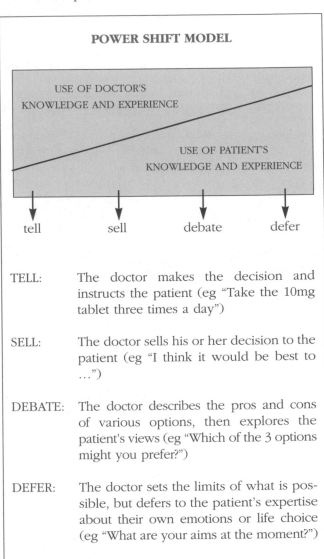

POWER SHIFT MODEL

USE OF DOCTOR'S
KNOWLEDGE AND EXPERIENCE

USE OF PATIENT'S
KNOWLEDGE AND EXPERIENCE

tell   sell   debate   defer

TELL: The doctor makes the decision and
           instructs the patient (eg "Take the 10mg
           tablet three times a day")

SELL: The doctor sells his or her decision to the
           patient (eg "I think it would be best to
           …")

DEBATE: The doctor describes the pros and cons
           of various options, then explores the
           patient's views (eg "Which of the 3 options
           might you prefer?")

DEFER: The doctor sets the limits of what is pos-
           sible, but defers to the patient's expertise
           about their own emotions or life choice
           (eg "What are your aims at the moment?")

(This model is also discussed briefly in Consultations I)

What is leadership?

A leader is defined as "a person who rules, guides or inspires others". A professional may inspire a patient to be more courageous, or more cheerful, or more trusting, and may therefore influence a patient's decisions indirectly. However, to directly guide or inspire a patient to make certain decisions is risky, because there is often an unequal distribution of power in a patient-professional relationship.

Does the patient want leadership?

Medical leadership is usually welcomed in an emergency (when time is short, consequences potentially serious, and no plan of action has been prepared). But should doctors provide leadership at other times? There has been a longstanding dispute about whether doctors should simply provide information and expertise (when they are sometimes accused of being "cold") or whether they should be warm and supportive (when others accuse them of being "patronizing"). Such arguments become redundant once it is realized that a spectrum of styles is needed, with different types of transaction being appropriate at different times (*see* Transactional Analysis).

What style of discussion is needed?

We need a variety of styles when talking with patients. The "power shift" model opposite shows how the involvement of the doctor (or other professional) can vary depending on the type of discussion the patient wants. Is a doctor-centered explanation of facts needed? (*see* Explanation). Or is a patient-centered discussion of emotions needed? (*see* Counselling). Or something in between?

Does the patient feel vulnerable or embarrassed?

When a patient meets a doctor there can be an unequal distribution of power and it can feel difficult or embarrassing for the patient to ask questions or admit to not understanding ("this will probably sound stupid, but ..."). The doctor has power in the form of information and being seen as a figure of authority. In addition in a hospital or hospice the environment is strange (and no-one is bigger than an organization). Some patients may also have experienced abusive relationships of unequal power in their past, and the consultation can re-awaken powerful memories or feelings of fear or anger. All these things can block decision-making.

How can the patient be empowered?

It may help the patient to make decisions if they feel more at ease and in control. There are 3 main ways that this happens. If the patient is allowed to: introduce or terminate new topics, tell their own story or to ask questions. To overcome embarrassment it can help to encourage questions: eg "Are there any things you want to ask about, even little things?".

LIVING WILLS

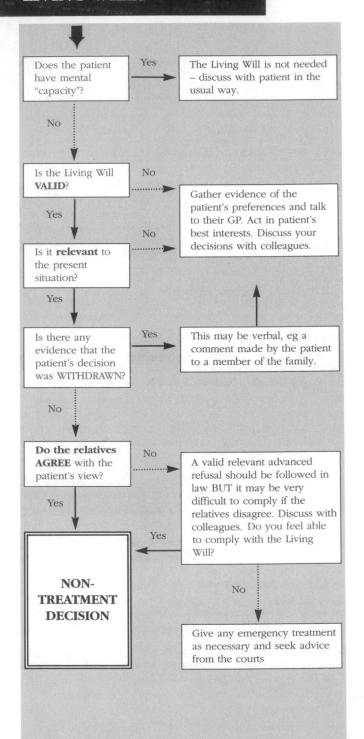

Does the patient have mental "capacity"? — **Yes** → The Living Will is not needed – discuss with patient in the usual way.

No

Is the Living Will **VALID**? — **No** ⇢

Yes

Is it **relevant** to the present situation? — **No** ⇢ Gather evidence of the patient's preferences and talk to their GP. Act in patient's best interests. Discuss your decisions with colleagues.

Yes

Is there any evidence that the patient's decision was WITHDRAWN? — **Yes** → This may be verbal, eg a comment made by the patient to a member of the family.

No

Do the relatives AGREE with the patient's view? — **No** ⇢ A valid relevant advanced refusal should be followed in law BUT it may be very difficult to comply if the relatives disagree. Discuss with colleagues. Do you feel able to comply with the Living Will?

Yes

NON-TREATMENT DECISION ← **Yes**

No ⇢ Give any emergency treatment as necessary and seek advice from the courts

144

What is a Living Will?

A Living Will is a document written when a patient is competent concerning preferences about medical treatment in the event of becoming incompetent. It is usually in effect an "advanced refusal of treatment" but a living will cannot oblige a doctor to <u>give</u> certain treatment. A general statement of preference is more useful than a lot of details because it is more likely to apply to a particular situation eg "If I become terminally ill with no likelihood of recovery, I want medical treatment to be limited to keeping me comfortable and I refuse all other medical treatment".

When should a Living Will become operative?

A Living Will is a communication tool to encourage early discussion of a patient's wishes about their future care. Ideally it will have been discussed several times already. The trigger for using an advanced directive usually occurs when an acute clinical event occurs in an unconscious patient. A junior hospital doctor who phoned me to ask "I have a patient dying on the ward and there is a Living Will in an envelope in the hospital notes, shall I open it yet?", had rather missed the point.

Can the patient change their mind?

A patient can obviously revoke a Living Will either verbally or in writing at any time.

When is a Living Will valid?

A Living Will is valid if at the time of signing it the patient had mental capacity, accurate information (did they see their GP?) and it was signed by a witness and it was never revoked (verbally or in writing) by the patient. Note that a lawyer need not be involved.

Is a Living Will legally binding?

A valid legal will is, legally binding (Just as if the patient had made a verbal request to refuse certain treatment) and it must not be ignored. A valid Living Will is enforceable by a court (and a decision made by a proxy appointed by the patient may also soon be enforceable in law in the UK).

What if the family disagree with a valid Living Will?

In this unfortunate situation it is usually best to give comfort care plus any emergency treatment and refer to the courts for advice.

What if the patient is obliged to receive treatment?

A patient receiving treatment under the Mental Health Act can still refuse any treatment not covered by the terms of their detention under the Act.

LYMPHOEDEMA

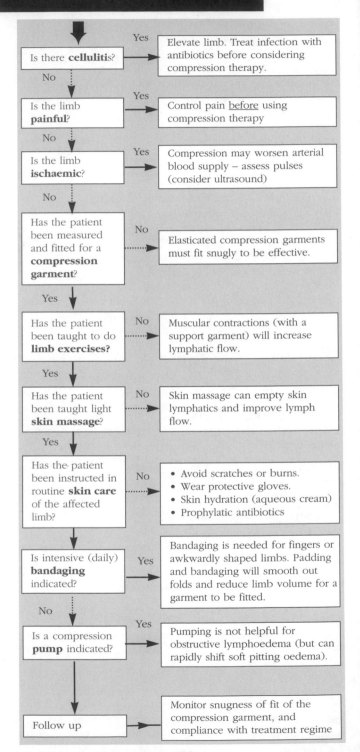

Is there cellulitis? — Yes → Elevate limb. Treat infection with antibiotics before considering compression therapy.

No ↓

Is the limb painful? — Yes → Control pain <u>before</u> using compression therapy

No ↓

Is the limb ischaemic? — Yes → Compression may worsen arterial blood supply – assess pulses (consider ultrasound)

No ↓

Has the patient been measured and fitted for a compression garment? — No → Elasticated compression garments must fit snugly to be effective.

Yes ↓

Has the patient been taught to do limb exercises? — No → Muscular contractions (with a support garment) will increase lymphatic flow.

Yes ↓

Has the patient been taught light skin massage? — No → Skin massage can empty skin lymphatics and improve lymph flow.

Yes ↓

Has the patient been instructed in routine skin care of the affected limb? — No →
- Avoid scratches or burns.
- Wear protective gloves.
- Skin hydration (aqueous cream)
- Prophylatic antibiotics

↓

Is intensive (daily) bandaging indicated? — Yes → Bandaging is needed for fingers or awkwardly shaped limbs. Padding and bandaging will smooth out folds and reduce limb volume for a garment to be fitted.

No ↓

Is a compression pump indicated? — Yes → Pumping is not helpful for obstructive lymphoedema (but can rapidly shift soft pitting oedema).

↓

Follow up → Monitor snugness of fit of the compression garment, and compliance with treatment regime

LYMPHOEDEMA

What is lymphoedema?
Lymphoedema means the swelling of the limb due to lymphatic obstruction. It causes a heavy and uncomfortable arm or leg, restricts movement and eventually causes skin thickening. An important part of management is teaching the patient and carer about control of the swelling. It can be hard for patients to realise that there is no cure and the management regime is "for life".

Is it a recent problem?
Recent onset lymphoedema is usually easier to shift. It is occasionally reversible (for a time) with high dose steroids.

Is there truncal oedema?
Oedema of the chest wall or abdomen can only be shifted by massage, and suggests a more severe problem.

How can massage help?
Stimulates lymph flow in the superficial lymph vessels which stimulates the normal lymphatic contractions and can milk lymph away from swollen area (massage starts in the <u>healthy</u> area and works towards the affected area). It must be demonstrated and taught properly.

Does the compression garment fit properly?
It is essential the support fits snugly. The patient's limb needs to be measured first. Good compression garments are made by Medi. Awkwardly-shaped limbs may need a special made-to-measure sleeve (eg Biersdorf).

Should exercises be recommended?
Limb exercise increases lymphatic flow, especially when using a compression garment and are an important part of management. Passive limb movements help if the patient is too weak to exercise.

Is bandaging necessary?
Bandaging with low pressure elastic bandages (eg secure 40) is useful for awkwardly-shaped limbs, finger swelling or lymphorrhoea.

Should a compression pump be used?
Compression pumps are not used routinely. They can be of benefit to rapidly clear soft oedema. They should be used at low pressure. They should not be used if there is trunk swelling. Sequential (multi-chamber) pumps are more effective than single chamber pumps.

Should diuretics be prescribed?
Diuretics are usually ineffective unless there is an element of venous obstruction and some pitting oedema superimposed on lymphoedema.

Is recurrent cellulitis a problem?
Damaged lymphatics are susceptible to infection, (which then cause further damage). Infection can be blood-born (ie can occur even without skin damage). Teach skin care and give pro-

MORPHINE 1 – USAGE

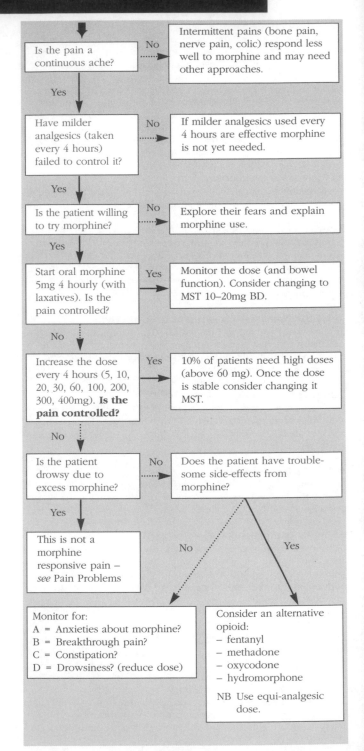

Is the pain a continuous ache? — No → Intermittent pains (bone pain, nerve pain, colic) respond less well to morphine and may need other approaches.

Yes ↓

Have milder analgesics (taken every 4 hours) failed to control it? — No → If milder analgesics used every 4 hours are effective morphine is not yet needed.

Yes ↓

Is the patient willing to try morphine? — No → Explore their fears and explain morphine use.

Yes ↓

Start oral morphine 5mg 4 hourly (with laxatives). Is the pain controlled? — Yes → Monitor the dose (and bowel function). Consider changing to MST 10–20mg BD.

No ↓

Increase the dose every 4 hours (5, 10, 20, 30, 60, 100, 200, 300, 400mg). **Is the pain controlled?** — Yes → 10% of patients need high doses (above 60 mg). Once the dose is stable consider changing it MST.

No ↓

Is the patient drowsy due to excess morphine? — No → Does the patient have troublesome side-effects from morphine?

Yes ↓

This is not a morphine responsive pain – *see* Pain Problems

No → Monitor for:
A = Anxieties about morphine?
B = Breakthrough pain?
C = Constipation?
D = Drowsiness? (reduce dose)

Yes → Consider an alternative opioid:
– fentanyl
– methadone
– oxycodone
– hydromorphone

NB Use equi-analgesic dose.

MORPHINE 1 – USAGE

When should morphine be started?
Morphine should be considered for any continuous pain that has not responded to other analgesics. Take a careful analgesic history before prescribing morphine – the doses of the analgesics used guide you about whether morphine is needed and also the correct starting dose, usually 5-10 mg 4 hourly, or 2.5 mg in the elderly or frail, or if it is for dyspnoea rather than for pain.

Is the patient frightened of using morphine?
Many patients (and families) fear that if you have cancer and morphine is prescribed it means "the beginning of the end" or the fear may be of addiction or of "becoming a zombie". Ask directly "Do you have any particular worries about taking morphine?" Explain that when used for pain (ie opioid-responsive pain) there is no danger of addiction, and even if taken for some time, stopping it may cause the pain to recur but will not cause "cold turkey" symptoms of goose-bumps, shivering, agitation etc. Similarly there is no danger of "becoming a zombie" if the dose is balanced carefully.

Does the patient understand the principles of balancing the dose?
It is important to spend some time explaining how the dose is monitored. If the pain persists then the regular dose is increased (but remains 4 hourly) but if the pain is controlled and the patient feels drowsy then the dose is reduced. Every day the patient needs to ask: "do I still have pain, am I feeling drowsy".

How often should the dose be changed?
On the first day the dose may need to be adjusted every 4 hours if the pain is not coming under control. For the next few days, it may only be necessary to adjust the dose every 24 hours or so. Once the dose is steady change over to a modified release morphine, with some immediate-release morphine for PRN use.

Is there fear about increasing the dose?
Some patients fear the dose going up "in case it no longer works when the pain gets very severe" or in case it means the disease is worsening and the end is nearing. Explain that there is no maximum dose, that the aim is to keep the patient free of pain, that there are no medals for suffering pain, that pain does not co-relate with disease progression and most importantly explain that the dose needed by each person is very individual, and needing a high dose may partly be due to a more efficient metabolism of morphine.

When should laxatives be started?
Almost every patient on morphine will get constipated (unless they already have a tendency to diarrhoea). Start laxatives on day 1, eg co-danthramer capsules 1-2 each night, and explain the "3 day rule": a suppository if no bowel movement for 3 days, and increase the daily laxative dose. The laxative dose may need to be increased if the morphine dose is increased.

How often should a patient on morphine be monitored?
Once the dose is steady and the patient is confident about how to use morphine, it is only necessary to see the patient every few weeks, telling them to ask for immediate advice if the pain control is lost.

See also: Morphine 2 – Preparations.

MORPHINE 2 – PREPARATIONS

Preparation	Frequency	Strength
ORAMORPH SOLUTION	4 hourly	• 10 mg/5 ml • 100 mg/5 ml • 5 ml oral vials (10, 30 100 mg)
SEVREDOL TABLETS	4 hourly	• 10 mg (blue) • 20 mg (pink) • 50 mg (green)
MST TABLETS OR SUSPENSION (Also effective via rectal route)	12 hourly	• 5 mg (white) • 10 mg (brown) • 15 mg (green) • 30 mg (purple) • 60 mg (orange) • 100 mg (grey) • 200 mg (green)
MXL CAPSULES	24 hourly	• 30 mg (light blue) • 60 mg (brown) • 90 mg (pink) • 120 mg (green) • 150 mg (blue) • 200 mg (orange)
MORCAP SR CAPSULES (contain pellets which can be sprinkled on food or given via gastrostomy tube)	24 hourly	• 20 mg (clear + 2 stripes) • 50 mg (clear + 3 stripes) • 100 mg (clear + 4 stripes)
ORAMORPH SR TABLETS	12 hourly	• 10 mg (brown) ie same • 30 mg (purple) colour-code • 60 mg (orange) as MST • 100 mg (grey)
ZOMORPH CAPSULES (contain pellets which can be sprinkled on food or given via gastrostomy tube)	12 hourly	• 10 mg (yellow/clear) • 30 mg (pink/clear) • 60 mg (orange/clear) • 100 mg (white/clear) • 200 mg (clear/clear)
CYCLIMORPH INJECTIONS (Best avoided)	PRN	• 10 mg • 15 mg Both have cyclizine 50 mg added. Too inflexible for adjusting morphine dose and cyclizine above 150 mg per day causes drowsiness.

MORPHINE 2 – PREPARATIONS

Which morphine preparation should be used?
It is usually best to start with a 4 hourly preparation until the optimum dose is established, then change to a longer-acting preparation.

Does the patient prefer liquids or tablets?
Use 4 hourly Oramorph solution if the patient has any problems swallowing tablets. Use 4 hourly Sevredol tablets if the patient prefers tablets (easier to carry around). The tablets are scored and can be broken in half.

When should modified-release morphine be used?
A modified-release form of morphine should be offered to all patients once a steady regular dose of 4 hourly morphine is achieved, because it simplifies the medication. A patient should **never** be prescribed more than one modified-release morphine at a time. Patients on slow-release morphine should **always** have some immediate release morphine for episodes of breakthrough pain.

What is the correct dose of PRN morphine for breakthrough pain?
The dose of morphine for breakthrough pain is the same as the regular 4 hrly morphine dose, eg if the patient is taking 30 mg Oramorph every 4 hours and develops some breakthrough pain they should take an extra 30 mg of Oramorph.

What should the patient be told about taking PRN morphine?
Extra morphine should be taken whenever the pain returns (if it is the same pain). There is no need to wait 4 hours. Even if the extra dose only lasts 1 hour, the patient should take another dose as soon as the pain becomes troublesome. A DIARY of PRN doses (date, time and dose) taken by the patient for a few days can be <u>very</u> helpful when first balancing the regular morphine dose.

MOUTH PROBLEMS

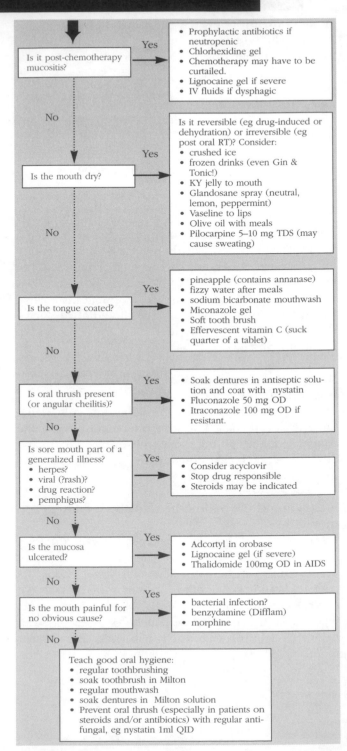

Is it post-chemotherapy mucositis? — Yes →
- Prophylactic antibiotics if neutropenic
- Chlorhexidine gel
- Chemotherapy may have to be curtailed.
- Lignocaine gel if severe
- IV fluids if dysphagic

No ↓

Is the mouth dry? — Yes →
Is it reversible (eg drug-induced or dehydration) or irreversible (eg post oral RT)? Consider:
- crushed ice
- frozen drinks (even Gin & Tonic!)
- KY jelly to mouth
- Glandosane spray (neutral, lemon, peppermint)
- Vaseline to lips
- Olive oil with meals
- Pilocarpine 5–10 mg TDS (may cause sweating)

No ↓

Is the tongue coated? — Yes →
- pineapple (contains annanase)
- fizzy water after meals
- sodium bicarbonate mouthwash
- Miconazole gel
- Soft tooth brush
- Effervescent vitamin C (suck quarter of a tablet)

No ↓

Is oral thrush present (or angular cheilitis)? — Yes →
- Soak dentures in antiseptic solution and coat with nystatin
- Fluconazole 50 mg OD
- Itraconazole 100 mg OD if resistant.

No ↓

Is sore mouth part of a generalized illness?
- herpes?
- viral (?rash)?
- drug reaction?
- pemphigus?
— Yes →
- Consider acyclovir
- Stop drug responsible
- Steroids may be indicated

No ↓

Is the mucosa ulcerated? — Yes →
- Adcortyl in orobase
- Lignocaine gel (if severe)
- Thalidomide 100mg OD in AIDS

No ↓

Is the mouth painful for no obvious cause? — Yes →
- bacterial infection?
- benzydamine (Difflam)
- morphine

No ↓

Teach good oral hygiene:
- regular toothbrushing
- soak toothbrush in Milton
- regular mouthwash
- soak dentures in Milton solution
- Prevent oral thrush (especially in patients on steroids and/or antibiotics) with regular anti-fungal, eg nystatin 1ml QID

Why is mouth care important?
A sore mouth is a very unpleasant symptom probably because the mouth has such a generous representation in the sensory cortex. 50–60% of hospice patients complain of a dry or sore mouth at some time, and it is the commonest symptom after general weakness. Oral hygiene can have a profound effect on a patients well-being "and a patients oral status is a very good index of general nursing care" (Crosby 1989).

Has the mouth been examined?
Examination of the mouth involves careful inspection, using a spatula a gloved finger and a pen torch. Inspect the roof of the mouth and inside the cheeks for evidence of thrush. If the mouth is dry or the tongue coated or shiny 4 hourly mouth care is needed. Malignant ulcers are often associated with anaerobic infections that produce a foul odour. This responds to metronidazole orally or rectally BD or as a topical gel.

Does the patient have dentures?
It is surprising how many patients with dentures keep them in over night. Dentures should be removed and soaked in a solution such as Milton's for at least 30 minutes (fungal hyphae can grow into the plastic of a denture plate). If thrush is a problem dentures can also can be coated with nystatin solution.

How often should routine mouth care be given?
Patients frequency of mouth care depends on the risk of mouth problems.

Low risk	–	4 hourly
Moderate risk	–	2 hourly
High risk	–	1 hourly

Risk factors include: chemotherapy, radiotherapy to the mouth, lethargy, drowsiness, low fluid intake, vomiting, weakness, dental decay, diabetes, steroids and dyspnoea.

Is it oral thrush? Thrush is a common feature of advanced illness, and made much more common by steroids or anti-biotics. The use of a systemic anti-fungal such as fluconazole 50mg daily has been a major advance in management, because it clears the infection so quickly. Nystatin 1 ml QID is mainly used as a preventive therapy in patients at high risk. Denture care is important (soak in Miltons, coat with nystatin). Resistant thrush usually responds to Itraconazole.

Is it a dental problem?
Dental caries or loose dentures should prompt referral to a dentist.

NAUSEA AND VOMITING

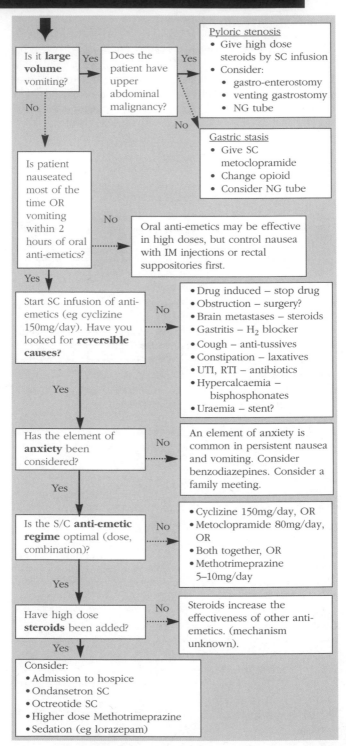

Is it **large volume** vomiting? — Yes → Does the patient have upper abdominal malignancy? — Yes →

Pyloric stenosis
- Give high dose steroids by SC infusion
- Consider:
  - gastro-enterostomy
  - venting gastrostomy
  - NG tube

No ↓

Gastric stasis
- Give SC metoclopramide
- Change opioid
- Consider NG tube

No ↓

Is patient nauseated most of the time OR vomiting within 2 hours of oral anti-emetics? — No →

Oral anti-emetics may be effective in high doses, but control nausea with IM injections or rectal suppositories first.

Yes ↓

Start SC infusion of anti-emetics (eg cyclizine 150mg/day). Have you looked for **reversible causes?** — No →

- Drug induced – stop drug
- Obstruction – surgery?
- Brain metastases – steroids
- Gastritis – H_2 blocker
- Cough – anti-tussives
- Constipation – laxatives
- UTI, RTI – antibiotics
- Hypercalcaemia – bisphosphonates
- Uraemia – stent?

Yes ↓

Has the element of **anxiety** been considered? — No →

An element of anxiety is common in persistent nausea and vomiting. Consider benzodiazepines. Consider a family meeting.

Yes ↓

Is the S/C **anti-emetic regime** optimal (dose, combination)? — No →

- Cyclizine 150mg/day, OR
- Metoclopramide 80mg/day, OR
- Both together, OR
- Methotrimeprazine 5–10mg/day

Yes ↓

Have high dose **steroids** been added? — No →

Steroids increase the effectiveness of other anti-emetics. (mechanism unknown).

Yes ↓

Consider:
- Admission to hospice
- Ondansetron SC
- Octreotide SC
- Higher dose Methotrimeprazine
- Sedation (eg lorazepam)

NAUSEA AND VOMITING

What is the cause?
Assessment (history, examination and tests) often reveals a potentially reversible cause (or causes). Treat with anti-emetics <u>simultaneously</u> with looking for and treating any underlying causes (eg infection, metabolic etc). If no cause is found it is probably due to tumour-related peptides (as yet unidentified).

Is it large volume vomiting?
This is usually due to malignant pyloric (high) obstruction, with projectile vomiting and often little preceding nausea. High dose steroids can reduce peri-tumour oedema and will "unblock" about 50%. A venting gastrostomy is a last resort but can stop vomiting and allow the patient to eat and drink normally (even though little is absorbed). An nasogastric tube should be a short-term measure but may allow a patient to get home. <u>Gastric stasis</u> causes reflux and heartburn as well as (<u>non</u>-projectile) vomiting and is often opioid-induced. Consider change of opioid.

Is the nausea controlled by oral anti-emetics?
Nausea causes gastric stasis. Oral anti-emetics may be poorly absorbed if there is nausea even without vomiting. Control nausea with IM\SC or PR drugs, and reserve oral anti-emetics for preventing recurrence.

Which anti-emetic?
The principle is to tailor the choice of anti-emetics to the likely cause of the nausea or vomiting. Although we are beginning to understand more about the receptor activity of these drugs, clinical practice is still largely based on experience, trial-and-error, and a limited logic:

Gastrokinetic	eg metoclopramide
Anticholinergic	eg cyclizine
Antidompaminergic	eg metoclopremide, haloperidol
5 HT3	eg ondansetron
Broad-spectrum	eg methotrimeprazine

30% of patients need more than one anti-emetic (and it is logical to combine drugs with different receptor activities).

Is it due to obstruction?
If surgery is not possible or appropriate the symptoms can be managed with a SC infusion of drugs. The aim is to abolish nausea, pain and colic. It may not be possible to abolish vomiting altogether in obstruction, but the patient can still eat and drink and most patients tolerate the occasional vomit well provided they are free of nausea (see Subcutaneous infusions).

Is nausea or vomiting difficult to control?
Monitor treatment by asking the patient to keep a DIARY of their symptoms, which helps analyse the pattern. It may be necessary to admit the patient for re-hydration, therapeutic trials or investigations. Quite often the symptom settles in the more secure environment of a hospice, suggesting anxiety is one component of the problem.

See also: Intestinal obstruction, Subcutaneous drugs, Subcutaneous infusions.

NUTRITION

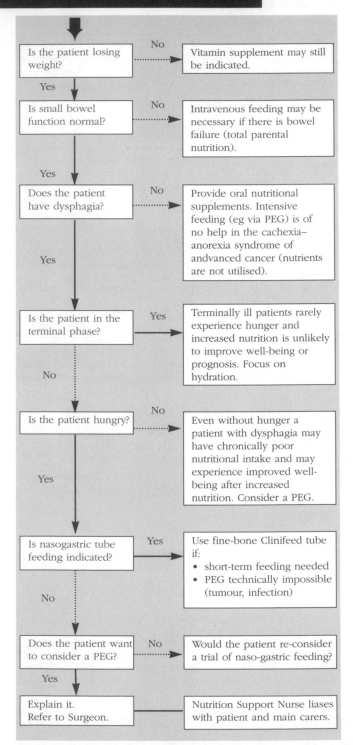

Is the patient losing weight? — No → Vitamin supplement may still be indicated.

Yes ↓

Is small bowel function normal? — No → Intravenous feeding may be necessary if there is bowel failure (total parental nutrition).

Yes ↓

Does the patient have dysphagia? — No → Provide oral nutritional supplements. Intensive feeding (eg via PEG) is of no help in the cachexia–anorexia syndrome of andvanced cancer (nutrients are not utilised).

Yes ↓

Is the patient in the terminal phase? — Yes → Terminally ill patients rarely experience hunger and increased nutrition is unlikely to improve well-being or prognosis. Focus on hydration.

No ↓

Is the patient hungry? — No → Even without hunger a patient with dysphagia may have chronically poor nutritional intake and may experience improved well-being after increased nutrition. Consider a PEG.

Yes ↓

Is nasogastric tube feeding indicated? — Yes → Use fine-bone Clinifeed tube if:
- short-term feeding needed
- PEG technically impossible (tumour, infection)

No ↓

Does the patient want to consider a PEG? — No → Would the patient re-consider a trial of naso-gastric feeding?

Yes ↓

Explain it. Refer to Surgeon. — Nutrition Support Nurse liases with patient and main carers.

156

When should a PEG be considered?

A PEG (percutaneous endoscopic gastrostomy) should be considered for any patient with dysphagia who is hungry or losing weight rapidly due to inadequate food intake.

Is a PEG useful for the cachexia-anorexia syndrome?

No. Increased nutrition does not cause weight gain or improve well-being or prognosis in this syndrome because the nutrients are not utilised (because there is a fundamental change to the metabolism).

Should early insertion of a PEG be considered?

A PEG is inserted endoscopically and early insertion may be considered in cancer of the throat or oesophagus if the disease is expected to progress to cause an obstruction. An open gastrostomy is a fairly simple operation and may be a reasonable alternative.

Is a PEG ever useful in partial dysphagia?

Yes. Patients with head and neck cancers may have many months of gradually increasing dysphagia, when they can still eat slowly but intake is inadequate and weight is gradually decreasing due to poor food intake rather than tumour progression. Dieticians often advocate an early PEG in this situation, before severe weight loss occurs, and the patient can still enjoy eating small amounts even with the PEG in place. It can be sensible to describe the option of a PEG early in the disease if dysphagia is likely to become a problem.

Has the patient and family had enough explanation?

A PEG is a small operation but a big decision for the patient, partly because eating is a social as well as a physiological activity. Discuss it carefully and more than once.

How is a PEG managed in the terminal phase?

In the terminal phase there is often a debate about how to reduce the feed via the PEG, in case the feeding is prolonging the dying phase. One solution is progressive dilution of the feed.

See also: Dysphagia, Hydration

ONCOLOGY DECISIONS

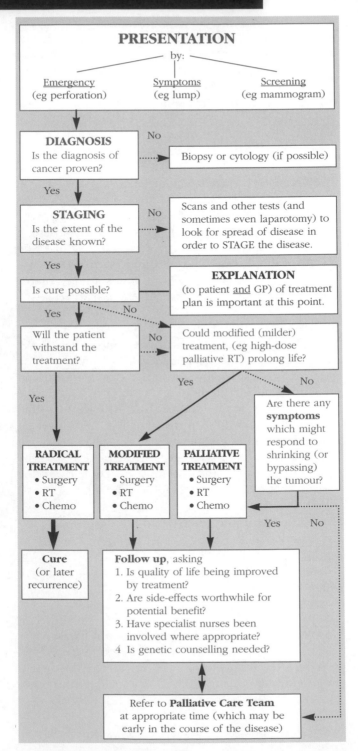

PRESENTATION
— by:

Emergency | Symptoms | Screening
(eg perforation) | (eg lump) | (eg mammogram)

DIAGNOSIS
Is the diagnosis of cancer proven? → No → Biopsy or cytology (if possible)

Yes ↓

STAGING
Is the extent of the disease known? → No → Scans and other tests (and sometimes even laparotomy) to look for spread of disease in order to STAGE the disease.

Yes ↓

Is cure possible? → **EXPLANATION** (to patient and GP) of treatment plan is important at this point.

Yes ↓ ⋯ No

Will the patient withstand the treatment? → No → Could modified (milder) treatment, (eg high-dose palliative RT) prolong life?

Yes ↓   Yes ↙   No ⋯→

Are there any **symptoms** which might respond to shrinking (or bypassing) the tumour?

RADICAL TREATMENT
• Surgery
• RT
• Chemo

MODIFIED TREATMENT
• Surgery
• RT
• Chemo

PALLIATIVE TREATMENT
• Surgery
• RT
• Chemo

Yes ← → No

Cure
(or later recurrence)

Follow up, asking
1. Is quality of life being improved by treatment?
2. Are side-effects worthwhile for potential benefit?
3. Have specialist nurses been involved where appropriate?
4 Is genetic counselling needed?

Refer to **Palliative Care Team** at appropriate time (which may be early in the course of the disease)

Has the diagnosis of cancer been proven?

The diagnosis of cancer may be strongly suspected from the history (eg pain and weight loss). Examination (eg a enlarged hard liver) or investigations (eg scans or raised plasma levels of tumour markers such as prostate specific antigen, PSA). However it is always best to have firm proof of diagnosis of cancer based on a tissue biopsy, which has been examined histologically to prove the presence of cancer cells (and to grade the level of aggressiveness of the cancer cells) prior to embarking on specific treatment for cancer.

Has the cancer spread?

It is important to stage the disease (ie to know the extent of the spread of the disease prior to planning treatment). Local disease is usually treated with surgery and or radiotherapy. Disease that is widespread is usually best treated with chemotherapy (unless local symptoms predominate).

Is cure possible?

It is important to explain the aims of treatment. If cure is not possible, explain this clearly from the beginning.

Has adequate explanation been given to the patient?

Once treatment is planned it is important that the patient understands both the aims of treatment and what the treatment programme will involve. It is also very important to explain this to the patients GP at this stage, so that the GP and the oncology department can work in harmony.

Is the oncology treatment helping or harming?

Long courses of radiotherapy or chemotherapy can produce side-effects as well as benefits, it is always a matter of judgement as to whether the benefits are out weighing the side-effects. This needs carefully re-assessing all the way through the treatment programme.

Should the palliative care team be involved?

Patients who are having particular difficulties, (physical or emotional) coping with the experience of illness may benefit from involvement of the multi-disciplinary palliative care team for symptom control or psychological support at any stage in a patient's oncology treatment. The palliative care team does not need to be reserved for terminally ill patients.

PAIN 1 – CONTROL

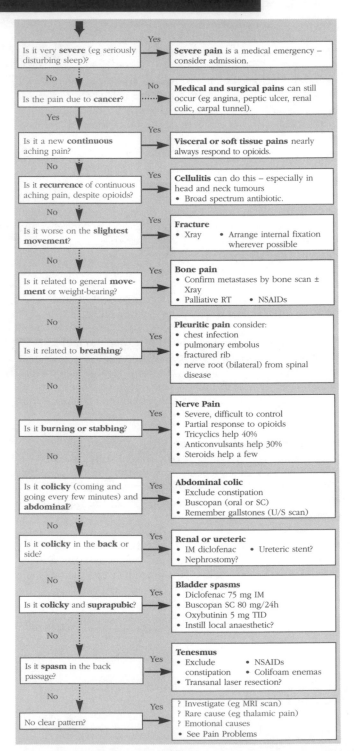

Is it very **severe** (eg seriously disturbing sleep)?	**Yes** →	**Severe pain** is a medical emergency – consider admission.
Is the pain due to **cancer**?	**No** ···→	**Medical and surgical pains** can still occur (eg angina, peptic ulcer, renal colic, carpal tunnel).
Is it a new **continuous** aching pain?	**Yes** →	**Visceral or soft tissue pains** nearly always respond to opioids.
Is it **recurrence** of continuous aching pain, despite opioids?	**Yes** →	**Cellulitis** can do this – especially in head and neck tumours • Broad spectrum antibiotic.
Is it worse on the **slightest movement**?	**Yes** →	**Fracture** • Xray • Arrange internal fixation wherever possible
Is it related to general **movement** or weight-bearing?	**Yes** →	**Bone pain** • Confirm metastases by bone scan ± Xray • Palliative RT • NSAIDs
Is it related to **breathing**?	**Yes** →	**Pleuritic pain** consider: • chest infection • pulmonary embolus • fractured rib • nerve root (bilateral) from spinal disease
Is it **burning or stabbing**?	**Yes** →	**Nerve Pain** • Severe, difficult to control • Partial response to opioids • Tricyclics help 40% • Anticonvulsants help 30% • Steroids help a few
Is it **colicky** (coming and going every few minutes) and **abdominal**?	**Yes** →	**Abdominal colic** • Exclude constipation • Buscopan (oral or SC) • Remember gallstones (U/S scan)
Is it **colicky** in the **back** or side?	**Yes** →	**Renal or ureteric** • IM diclofenac • Ureteric stent? • Nephrostomy?
Is it **colicky** and **suprapubic**?	**Yes** →	**Bladder spasms** • Diclofenac 75 mg IM • Buscopan SC 80 mg/24h • Oxybutinin 5 mg TID • Instill local anaesthetic?
Is it **spasm** in the back passage?	**Yes** →	**Tenesmus** • Exclude constipation • NSAIDs • Colifoam enemas • Transanal laser resection?
No clear pattern?	**Yes** →	? Investigate (eg MRI scan) ? Rare cause (eg thalamic pain) ? Emotional causes • See Pain Problems

This flow-chart is about routine methods of pain control for cancer pain. 30% of patients with cancer do not get cancer pain.

How should I assess pain?
Most pains are diagnosed from the pattern described by the patient. Ask about:

P = Place?
A = Analgesics tried?
R = Relation to movement?
T = Timing?
N = Nights and sleep?
E = Exacerbating factors?
R = Relieving factors?
S = Severity (0–10)?

Is it cancer pain?
Careful assessment (especially history-taking) is the key to good management. A simple example: A patient with liver metastases may have abdominal pains and may be started on morphine on the assumption that the pain is cancer pain. However the liver metastases may be pain free and the pain may be colicky pain due to constipation (which will be worsened by the morphine). It is essential to explore the pattern of each pain and to be on the look-out for non-cancer pain.

How should I assess cancer pain?
The patient's verbal report of the pain, which usually gives a clear indication of the type of cancer pain: <u>Continuous</u> pain (visceral or soft tissue) usually responds well to morphine. Pain <u>on movement</u> (bone pain) responds poorly to morphine, but is usually controlled by radiotherapy or NSAIDs. <u>Stabbing or burning</u> pain (nerve pain) responds partially to morphine, but usually needs tricyclics or anti-convulsants as well. <u>Colicky</u> pain that comes and goes may be due to treatable constipation or may respond to an anti-spasmodic, such as Buscopan.

Is the treatment controlling the pain?
<u>PAIN SCORES</u> are an effective and simple way to monitor pain control. The patient is asked 3 times a day to rate the severity of pain on a score of 0–10, where 0 is no pain at all and 10 is the worst pain imaginable. The scores are recorded on a chart. Uncontrolled pain needs re-assessment.

<u>See also</u> Analgesia, Fentanyl, Morphine, Pain Problems.

PAIN 2 – PROBLEMS

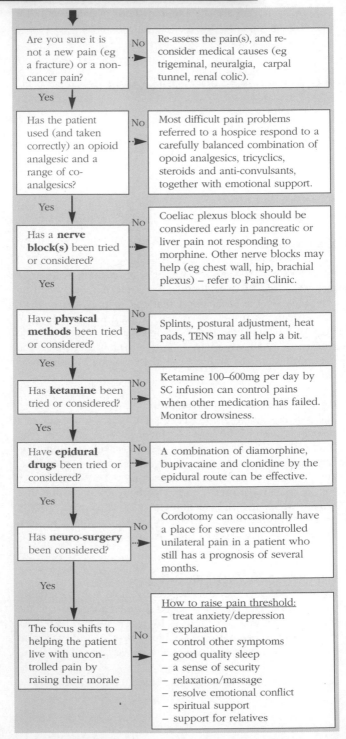

Are you sure it is not a new pain (eg a fracture) or a non-cancer pain? — **No** → Re-assess the pain(s), and re-consider medical causes (eg trigeminal, neuralgia, carpal tunnel, renal colic).

Yes ↓

Has the patient used (and taken correctly) an opioid analgesic and a range of co-analgesics? — **No** → Most difficult pain problems referred to a hospice respond to a carefully balanced combination of opoid analgesics, tricyclics, steroids and anti-convulsants, together with emotional support.

Yes ↓

Has a **nerve block(s)** been tried or considered? — **No** → Coeliac plexus block should be considered early in pancreatic or liver pain not responding to morphine. Other nerve blocks may help (eg chest wall, hip, brachial plexus) – refer to Pain Clinic.

Yes ↓

Have **physical methods** been tried or considered? — **No** → Splints, postural adjustment, heat pads, TENS may all help a bit.

Yes ↓

Has **ketamine** been tried or considered? — **No** → Ketamine 100–600mg per day by SC infusion can control pains when other medication has failed. Monitor drowsiness.

Yes ↓

Have **epidural drugs** been tried or considered? — **No** → A combination of diamorphine, bupivacaine and clonidine by the epidural route can be effective.

Yes ↓

Has **neuro-surgery** been considered? — **No** → Cordotomy can occasionally have a place for severe uncontrolled unilateral pain in a patient who still has a prognosis of several months.

Yes ↓

The focus shifts to helping the patient live with uncon-trolled pain by raising their morale — **No** → How to raise pain threshold:
– treat anxiety/depression
– explanation
– control other symptoms
– good quality sleep
– a sense of security
– relaxation/massage
– resolve emotional conflict
– spiritual support
– support for relatives

This flow chart is about difficult pain problems which do not respond to routine measures (about 5% of cancer pains). Difficult pains are commonly due to nerve damage ("neuropathic pain").

Have I re-assessed the pain?
The pain may have changed. Is it the same pain as before, or has a new pain occurred? Are there 2 different pains occuring together which need different treatments?

Is the patient taking their medication correctly?
This is a common cause of uncontrolled pain. Re-assess the prescribed medicines and exactly how they are being taken.

Have I re-assessed the management?
Has every option been explored? Should the patient be referred back to the oncologist to re-consider further RT or chemotherapy? Are further investigations needed to seek a cause for the pain, eg MRI scan.

Has a pain DIARY been kept?
A pain diary is a very useful way of understanding the pattern of the pain more clearly and seeing which medications are most helpful. Ask the patient to write notes through the day of when the pain is bad, what they were doing and action taken, then analyse it carefully with them. A pain diary should not be kept for more than a week or so, because it can increase the patient's focus on the pain and can become demoralising.

Are there any other drugs which should be tried?
Ketamine has been shown to control some pains unresponsive to other analgesics. Are you up-to-date with new treatment options? Have you discussed this pain problem with other palliative medicine specialists?

Is referral to the pain clinic indicated?
Discuss the problem with your local pain clinic or Anaesthetist specialising in pain control. A nerve block or epidural infusion of analgesics can help control some difficult pains. Seek advice before assuming there is nothing to offer.

Is emotional distress worsening the pain?
Pain is made worse by emotional distress. Also, sometimes, emotional distress presents as a physical pain that cannot be controlled (which has been called "opioid-irrelevant" pain). Any severe pain has to be managed by focusing on both the physical and emotional elements of the pain. What is the meaning of the pain (eg "does it mean the cancer is spreading?"). Who else is it affecting? What is it stopping the patient from doing? What does the patient do when the pain is severe? Are there any emotional or family difficulties making it more difficult to cope with this pain?

PALLIATIVE CARE

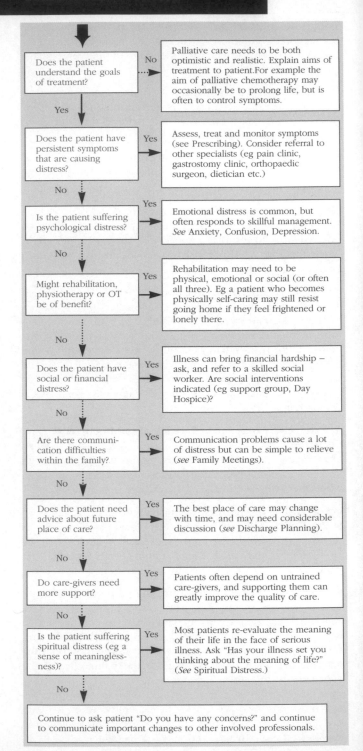

Does the patient understand the goals of treatment? — No → Palliative care needs to be both optimistic and realistic. Explain aims of treatment to patient. For example the aim of palliative chemotherapy may occasionally be to prolong life, but is often to control symptoms.

Yes ↓

Does the patient have persistent symptoms that are causing distress? — Yes → Assess, treat and monitor symptoms (see Prescribing). Consider referral to other specialists (eg pain clinic, gastrostomy clinic, orthopaedic surgeon, dietician etc.)

No ↓

Is the patient suffering psychological distress? — Yes → Emotional distress is common, but often responds to skillful management. *See* Anxiety, Confusion, Depression.

No ↓

Might rehabilitation, physiotherapy or OT be of benefit? — Yes → Rehabilitation may need to be physical, emotional or social (or often all three). Eg a patient who becomes physically self-caring may still resist going home if they feel frightened or lonely there.

No ↓

Does the patient have social or financial distress? — Yes → Illness can bring financial hardship – ask, and refer to a skilled social worker. Are social interventions indicated (eg support group, Day Hospice)?

No ↓

Are there communication difficulties within the family? — Yes → Communication problems cause a lot of distress but can be simple to relieve (*see* Family Meetings).

No ↓

Does the patient need advice about future place of care? — Yes → The best place of care may change with time, and may need considerable discussion (*see* Discharge Planning).

No ↓

Do care-givers need more support? — Yes → Patients often depend on untrained care-givers, and supporting them can greatly improve the quality of care.

No ↓

Is the patient suffering spiritual distress (eg a sense of meaninglessness)? — Yes → Most patients re-evaluate the meaning of their life in the face of serious illness. Ask "Has your illness set you thinking about the meaning of life?" (*See* Spiritual Distress.)

No ↓

Continue to ask patient "Do you have any concerns?" and continue to communicate important changes to other involved professionals.

PALLIATIVE CARE

What is Palliative Care?

Palliative Care is defined by The World Health Organisation as "The active total care of patients who's disease is not responsive to curative treatment". The aim of palliative care is to promote the comfort and quality of life of the patient, without prolonging or hastening death and to support the patients family. It is characterised by a multi-disciplinary team approach to care and by high quality communication both with the patient and family, and also between professionals. Palliative Care can be delivered in a hospital setting (with or without dedicated beds) the home, a hospice or the nursing home.

When should the specialist palliative care team be involved?

Many patients with malignant and non-malignant conditions benefit from a palliative care approach. Palliative care is needed at times in almost all medical and surgical specialities. A specialist palliative care team can be used as a resource at any stage of illness, if there are difficult or uncontrolled symptoms or if the patient and family need intensive emotional support. A palliative care team need not take over care and does not need to be reserved for terminally ill patients.

Does the patient understand the concept of palliative care?

Patients can be confused about what "palliative" means eg the difference between radical (curative) radiotherapy and palliative radiotherapy often needs careful explanation. Patients can also be confused about what palliative care has to offer them. It can help to explain that the focus is helping them and their families to cope with the experience of being ill, rather than focusing mainly on the disease process.

How is a patient cared for by a team?

A multi-diciplinary team can be a very effective way of providing care to a patient and family when they have complex needs in a changing situation. However, team work can also lead to problems if there is poor communication within the team or if patients get conflicting advice from team members. It can also be difficult for a sick patient to relate to large numbers of new faces and to re-tell their story many times. It is important to try and rationalise the number of professionals involved. This can be achieved by team members accepting some role over lap and supporting each other behind the scenes.

See also: Assessment.

PERSONALITY TYPES

4 SCALES OF PERSONALITY

Each scale measures
Preferences
For a different
Aspect of personality

⇩

Extrovert (E) ------- Gaining energy ------ **Introvert** (I)

Sensing (S) ------ Taking in information --- i**N**tuitive (N)

Thinking (T) ---------- Deciding ---------- **Feeling** (F)

Judging (J --------------- Acting ----------- **Perceiving** (P)

E	**Extrovert types** – prefer to focus on people and things, and tend to act before thinking.	I	**Introvert types** – prefer to focus on ideas and impressions and may think so much that they fail to act.
S	**Sensing types** prefer established routines and are organised and precise. They tend to see the objections to new ideas before the good points.	N	**iNtuitive types** – like solving new problems, and can often see what "could be" but tend to jump to conclusions and ignore the practical details.
T	**Thinking types** prefer to base decisions on logic and analysis, and can seem impersonal, and tend to ignore people's feelings, including their own.	F	**Feeling types** prefer to base decisions on feelings and can get upset by arguments. Good at assessing the human consequences of decisions, but may postpone tough decisions in an attempt to maintain harmony.
J	**Judging types** prefer to act according to plans and schedules. They tend to make lists. They can be reluctant to move from or question given values. They can come to a decision too quickly, and then ignore the evidence to the contrary. May be over-respectful of authority.	P	**Perceiving types** prefer to act spontaneously. They tend to be good at adapting to change, but often have difficulty making final decisions because they always want to consider more information.

	Sensing types		Intuitive types	
Intravert types	**IS**TJ	**IS**FJ	**IN**FJ	**IN**TJ
	ISTP	**IS**FP	**IN**FP	**IN**TP
Extravert types	**ES**TP	**ES**FP	**EN**FP	**EN**TP
	ESTJ	**ES**FJ	**EN**FJ	**EN**TJ

Can personality be assessed?

The Myers-Briggs method is a popular way of describing personality differences. It uses 4 scales to look at 4 different aspects of personality:

- how we prefer to recover our energy (from others or from within ourselves)
- how we prefer to perceive stimuli
- how we prefer to decide
- how we prefer to act.

It is not about what is "normal" but about preferences and differences.

How do personality types differ?

The boxes opposite describe the characteristics of each end of the 4 scales (with particular reference to decision-making styles). Note that it is about preferences. Most people have some characteristics at both ends of each scale, but will prefer one end to the other. To find your own personality type see which end of each scale you prefer (when you are relaxed and "being yourself"). A more detailed questionnaire is needed to be sure which end of the scale you prefer.

How does personality affect decisions?

People vary in the ways they prefer to take in new information and make decisions. For example, a person who is ENFP (ie who prefers those ends of the 4 scales) may like to take risks, whereas a person who is ISTJ may be risk aversive.

How does understanding personality help?

It helps to be aware of your own preferences when making decisions. Approaches that you may tend to neglect, may be useful for a particular problem. Also, patients may think very differently to you. For example, if you are an ESTJ you may see a particular decision as straightforward, and may find it very difficult to understand or tolerate the relatively off-the-wall decision-making approach of a patient who is an INFP! The main valve of understanding personality types is that it reminds us how much people can differ.

Can personality change?

Yes – a person may change their preference, especially if a major change occurs in life-style, eg through serious illness. Ask about the patient's previous personality.

PRESCRIBING

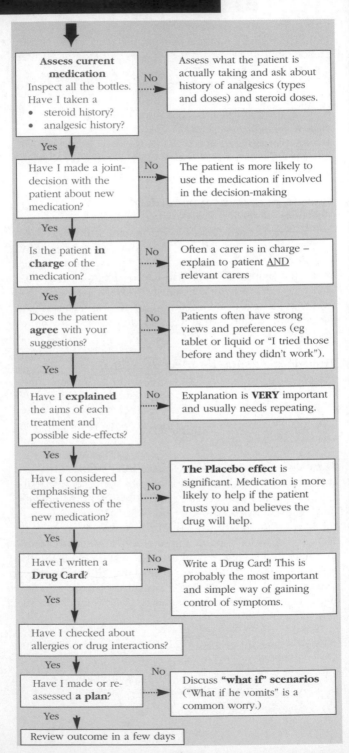

Assess current medication
Inspect all the bottles.
Have I taken a
- steroid history?
- analgesic history?

No ····▶ Assess what the patient is actually taking and ask about history of analgesics (types and doses) and steroid doses.

Yes ▼

Have I made a joint-decision with the patient about new medication?

No ····▶ The patient is more likely to use the medication if involved in the decision-making

Yes ▼

Is the patient **in charge** of the medication?

No ····▶ Often a carer is in charge – explain to patient <u>AND</u> relevant carers

Yes ▼

Does the patient **agree** with your suggestions?

No ····▶ Patients often have strong views and preferences (eg tablet or liquid or "I tried those before and they didn't work").

Yes ▼

Have I **explained** the aims of each treatment and possible side-effects?

No ····▶ Explanation is **VERY** important and usually needs repeating.

Yes ▼

Have I considered emphasising the effectiveness of the new medication?

No ····▶ **The Placebo effect** is significant. Medication is more likely to help if the patient trusts you and believes the drug will help.

Yes ▼

Have I written a **Drug Card**?

No ····▶ Write a Drug Card! This is probably the most important and simple way of gaining control of symptoms.

Yes ▼

Have I checked about allergies or drug interactions?

Yes ▼

Have I made or re-assessed **a plan**?

No ····▶ Discuss **"what if" scenarios** ("What if he vomits" is a common worry.)

Yes ▼

Review outcome in a few days

168

What medication is the patient already taking?
Find out what the patient is already <u>actually</u> taking (and how often). Do not assume that everything is being taken exactly as prescribed. Also, find out what has been tried in the past (eg what analgesics?).

What drug shall I prescribe?
What is most likely to help the patient the most without causing unacceptable side-effects? Would an alternative drug help more? Have I considered interactions with other drugs being taken? Have I asked about allergies? Is the outcome of using this drug uncertain? Should I discuss the uncertainties? Who will monitor it? For how long will it need to be continued?

Will the patient accept it?
Has the patient tried it before? Will they consider it? Have they established enough trust in the prescriber? Does the patient have strong preferences eg liquid medication but not tablets? Do any of the close relatives object to the drug, and might they persuade the patient not to take it.

Has the best route been considered?
The best route may be oral, IM, suppository, inhaled, transdermal or SC infusion. Is the patient getting tired of swallowing a lot of medication?

Has enough explanation been given?
Does the patient (and carer) understand the aim of the treatment, and how the drug works? Most drugs have side-effects, some more important than others. Is the patient concerned about side-effects? Which side-effects should be mentioned?

Has a drug card been written?
A drug card is a simple communication tool which is a highly effective way of improving symptom control. It clarifies the names of the medication (which often causes confusion) and it explains what they are all for, and when to take them. Debate the best times (eg "What time do you normally take tablets in the morning?"). Find out who is in charge of the medication. It is usually best to explain the chart to both the patient and the main carer.

DRUG	TIMES 9am	1pm	5pm	9pm	PURPOSE
MST	1			1	Pain
Co-danthramer				1	Laxative
Metoclopramide	1	1	1	1	Nausea

Can any medication be stopped?
Drugs can be stopped as well as started. If drugs have not helped stop them. Some long-term medication may no longer be appropriate, eg anti-hypertensive drugs can often be reduced or stopped in patients who have lost a lot of weight, because their blood pressure may now be in the normal range. Stopping long-term medication usually needs careful explanation.

PRESSURE SORES

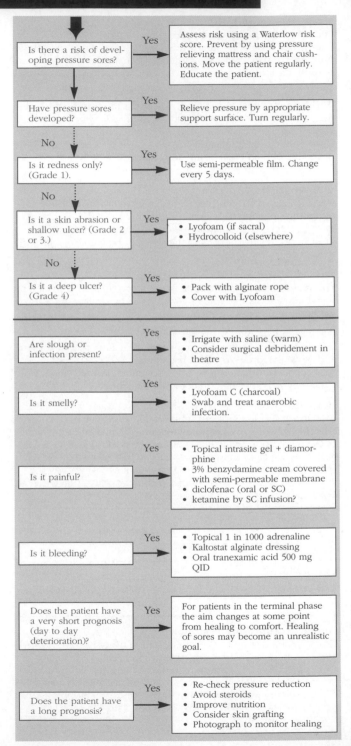

Is there a risk of developing pressure sores? — **Yes** → Assess risk using a Waterlow risk score. Prevent by using pressure relieving mattress and chair cushions. Move the patient regularly. Educate the patient.

Have pressure sores developed? — **Yes** → Relieve pressure by appropriate support surface. Turn regularly.

No

Is it redness only? (Grade 1). — **Yes** → Use semi-permeable film. Change every 5 days.

No

Is it a skin abrasion or shallow ulcer? (Grade 2 or 3.) — **Yes** →
- Lyofoam (if sacral)
- Hydrocolloid (elsewhere)

No

Is it a deep ulcer? (Grade 4) — **Yes** →
- Pack with alginate rope
- Cover with Lyofoam

Are slough or infection present? — **Yes** →
- Irrigate with saline (warm)
- Consider surgical debridement in theatre

Is it smelly? — **Yes** →
- Lyofoam C (charcoal)
- Swab and treat anaerobic infection.

Is it painful? — **Yes** →
- Topical intrasite gel + diamorphine
- 3% benzydamine cream covered with semi-permeable membrane
- diclofenac (oral or SC)
- ketamine by SC infusion?

Is it bleeding? — **Yes** →
- Topical 1 in 1000 adrenaline
- Kaltostat alginate dressing
- Oral tranexamic acid 500 mg QID

Does the patient have a very short prognosis (day to day deterioration)? — **Yes** → For patients in the terminal phase the aim changes at some point from healing to comfort. Healing of sores may become an unrealistic goal.

Does the patient have a long prognosis? — **Yes** →
- Re-check pressure reduction
- Avoid steroids
- Improve nutrition
- Consider skin grafting
- Photograph to monitor healing

Is the patient at risk?
Prevention is better than cure. It is especially important to institute pressure relieving regimes where a patient is at increased risk of developing pressure sores. The main risk factors are:

RISK FACTORS

– age	– radiotherapy
– immobility	– anaemia
– poor nutritional status	– chemotherapy
– cachexia	– incontinence
– steroid therapy	

What are risk scales?
There are various risk assessment tools (eg Waterlow) but it is unclear how accurate they are or whether they improve outcome. Clinical judgement is just as important. What is especially effective is developing a protocol for standardised care and having a team member with a special interest in prevention and treatment of pressure sores.

How should high risk patients be nursed?
Patients with pressure sores, or those at high risk should be nursed on low pressure (or alternating pressure) mattresses. These have been shown to be more effective than standard hospital beds. However which type of specialised support service is best remains a matter of opinion and no clinical trials exist. The manual handling skills of the nursing team are particularly important. Lateral shearing forces on the skin when a patient is moved can rapidly produce pressure sores, as can constant exposure to low pressure.

How often should patients be assessed?
A patient should be assessed for pressure area care within 2 hours of admission, again at 48 hours and then weekly or if their condition worsens.

How often should a patient be turned?
Effectiveness of different schedules of manual repositioning has not been adequately studied. Current best practice is to turn 2 hourly. Changing the patient's position by a 30 degree tilt relieves pressure as effectively as complete turning.

What is the aim of treatment?
Once pressure sores have developed the aim is usually to heal them as quickly as possible. The most important factor for healing is relief of pressure. For patients in the terminal phase the aim changes at some point from healing to comfort. Trying to maximise comfort may alter decisions about how often dressings are changed or the patient is moved.

What is the best dressing?
Modern dressings promote moist wound healing, and have been a useful advance, but the best ones still remain a matter of opinion and experience – the flow chart opposite gives a guide to acceptable practice.

PROBABILITY

USING THE LOTTERY TO EXPLAIN RISK

The lottery is one way of helping patients to understand probabilities and relative risks. It helps explain the concept of "doubling of risk", which is like doubling your stake from £5 to £10. This increases your chance of getting 3 numbers to 1 in 5 (about once a month on a weekly gamble), whereas your chance of getting 6 numbers would still only be once every 29,000 years! In other words, for a relatively common event doubling of risk is significant to an individual, but for a relatively rare event it is not. In otherwords double a very remote risk and you still have a very remote risk.

RISK OF WINNING THE LOTTERY FOR A £5 STAKE

Number of Balls	Probability Scale	Verbal Scale
3	1:10	High
4	1:200	Moderate
5	1:11,000	Very low
5 + bonus	1:500,000	Minimal
6	1:3,000,000	Negligible

For a £5 stake once a week, you should get 3 balls correct (and win £10) once every 14 weeks, and 6 balls correct (and win the jackpot) once every 3 million weeks (58,000 years!)

What does "doubling of risk" mean?

The recent "pill scare" led to thousands of unwanted pregnancies, because many women stopped their pill suddenly when the media emphasised that the risk of thrombosis had doubled with the new pill being precribed. But the risk of thrombosis was so small (1.5 deaths per million women years) that doubling the risk meant that there was still a negligible risk to an individual (still only 3 deaths per million women years). The absolute risk had doubled, but the relative risk was still very low, because it is so rare in the first place. Similarly if a treatment leads to a reduction in risk of 50% it may be significant for a patient at high risk, but not for patients at low risk, because the size of the risk reduction might not be sufficient to warrant the toxicity or cost of the treatment.

What is risk?

Risk means there are various possible outcomes, with known probabilities (whereas uncertainty means that the probabilities are unknown). Many clinical decisions involve risk, and therefore involve probabilities. Patients need to be given information about probability in a form they can understand.

What is Probability?

Probability is a statistical concept. In scientific papers probability is described as a p number or as a %. We often use p=0.05 (or a 5% chance) as an artificial cut-off point: if A causes B with a probability of p=0.05 it means that the probability that it occurred by chance is only 5% or 1 in 20 (or 1 in 100 if p=0.01).

Is the probability known?

In medicine we are often dealing with uncertainties. when probabilities are not known, and we have to make decisions based on "probable cause", "weight of evidence" and "reasonable doubt". In fact when we talk of "probability" we often really mean a non-mathematical concept of "the degree of belief warranted by the information just presented".

How relevant are the statistics?

Statistics derived from a group may not apply to an individual (who belongs to that group but who also belongs to lots of other groups). For example, knowing that the median survival after diagnosis of mesothelioma is only 8 months, tells you nothing about the probability of the patient being in the 5% who survive several years.

What is "number needed to treat"?

The benefits of treatment are often described in terms of a relative risk reduction, expressed as a %, but the number needed to treat (the inverse of the absolute risk reduction) can be a more helpful figure for both the doctor and the patient. For example 2 groups of hypertensive patients may both have a relative risk reduction (for having a stroke) of 40% for a particular treatment, suggesting both should be treated equally vigorously. But the number needed to treat (to prevent 1 stroke every 5 years) is 13 for moderate hypertension, but 167 for mild hypertension, suggesting the clinical recommendations are likely to be different for the 2 groups. Similarly the risk of side-effects from a particular treatment can be described in terms of "number needed to harm".

PROBLEM SOLVING

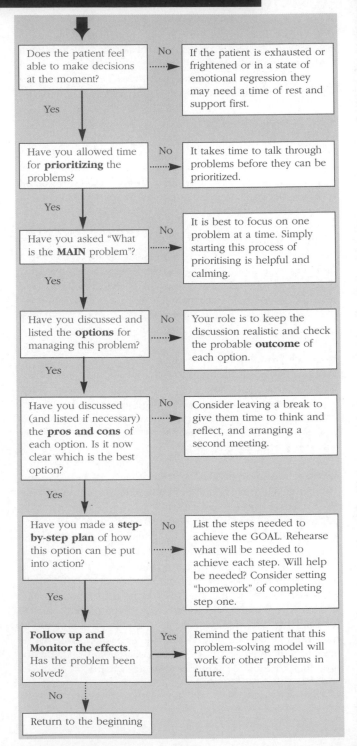

Does the patient feel able to make decisions at the moment?

No → If the patient is exhausted or frightened or in a state of emotional regression they may need a time of rest and support first.

Yes

Have you allowed time for **prioritizing** the problems?

No → It takes time to talk through problems before they can be prioritized.

Yes

Have you asked "What is the **MAIN** problem"?

No → It is best to focus on one problem at a time. Simply starting this process of prioritising is helpful and calming.

Yes

Have you discussed and listed the **options** for managing this problem?

No → Your role is to keep the discussion realistic and check the probable **outcome** of each option.

Yes

Have you discussed (and listed if necessary) the **pros and cons** of each option. Is it now clear which is the best option?

No → Consider leaving a break to give them time to think and reflect, and arranging a second meeting.

Yes

Have you made a **step-by-step plan** of how this option can be put into action?

No → List the steps needed to achieve the GOAL. Rehearse what will be needed to achieve each step. Will help be needed? Consider setting "homework" of completing step one.

Yes

Follow up and Monitor the effects. Has the problem been solved?

Yes → Remind the patient that this problem-solving model will work for other problems in future.

No

Return to the beginning

What is problem-solving?

Problem-solving is a useful technique in palliative care, when used in addition to general support and counselling.

It is a simple, brief psychological treatment based on the common observation that emotional symptoms often relate to practical and social problems of daily living.

It is a simple (teachable) method of helping patients (and ourselves!) to make decisions. Teaching a simple method of problem solving is especially useful when patients feel confused and overwhelmed by having to make decisions. Simply starting the process often has a calming effect. Problem-solving involves 5 stages (which do not need to happen on the same day).

1. List problems – then select <u>main</u> one.

2. List options (for dealing with <u>main</u> problem).

3. Look at pros and cons of each option.

4. Select best option.

5. Make a <u>plan of action</u> divided into simple <u>manageable steps</u>. Help the patient tackle step one. Monitor results.

A good way of considering the pros and cons of various options is by the "Jesuit cross":

<u>CONSIDERING PROS AND CONS</u>	
<u>Advantages</u> of having the operation	<u>Advantages</u> of NOT having the operation
<u>Disadvantages</u> of having the operation	<u>Disadvantages</u> of NOT having the operation

Once the pros and cons are listed and considered the best option often becomes clear.

Is "homework" appropriate?

Suggesting a written "task", to be discussed later can be helpful. The patient may need some *time* to list or prioritize problems, or to consider the pros and cons of different options.

See also: Crisis Intervention

WHAT SORT OF QUESTION SHOULD I ASK NEXT?

Do you have any pain?	What do you understand about your illness?	What are you unable to do at the moment?	What is the hardest thing for you at the moment?	How do you feel about what we have just discussed?	How is this illness affecting your family?
(A closed question inviting a 'yes' or 'no' answer to focus the conversation)					

THE CONVERSATION BECOMES

| Disease orientated | Insight orientated | Illness orientated | Person orientated | Empathy orientated | Family orientated |

What questions should we ask?
When talking with patients we frequently have to make (internal) decisions about what question to ask. These decisions are important because as professionals our questions powerfully influence the direction of the consultation (see chart opposite). The quality of our shared decision-making with a patient relates to the quality of our questions.

Are any type of questions <u>un</u>helpful?
Avoid <u>leading</u> questions (eg "Are you well, today?") which lead the patient to a particular response. Avoid <u>multiple</u> questions, because asking more than one thing at once is confusing.

What are "open questions"?
Open questions start with "What", "Why" or "How" and tend to open up the conversation and encourage a patient to talk about their concerns and feelings. Most of our questions should be open questions. Closed questions ("do you" ,"have you", "are you") invite a reply of either "yes" or "no" which can be useful to keep a very talkative patient to the point.

What are "hypothetical questions"?
Hypothetical questions start with "If——" and are very useful for exploring patient's concerns, and for asking questions about sensitive topics, eg "IF the time comes for you to need more nursing help, would you want to be cared for at home?"

What does "interlacing" mean?
Interlacing means asking questions about feelings from time to time throughout any conversation, eg How do you feel about what I just said?

What are reflective questions?
Reflective questions (reflecting the question or comment back to the patient) are useful for handling difficult questions, (eg "I am wondering what made you ask that question at this particular moment?") for exploring how much information a patient wants, (eg "You mentioned being "in the dark", would it help you to have a bit more information about your illness?") and for exploring feelings in more depth, (eg "When you said "devastated" What did you mean?")

Does the patient have any questions?
Questions steer the direction of a conversation. It can empower patients to be involved with decision-making if they are allowed or encouraged to ask questions.

See also: Leadership

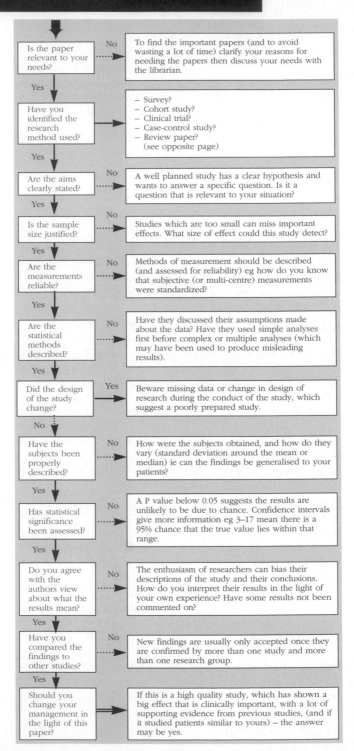

| Is the paper relevant to your needs? | No ┈┈▶ | To find the important papers (and to avoid wasting a lot of time) clarify your reasons for needing the papers then discuss your needs with the librarian. |

Yes ▼

| Have you identified the research method used? | ▶ | – Survey?
– Cohort study?
– Clinical trial?
– Case-control study?
– Review paper?
(see opposite page) |

Yes ▼

| Are the aims clearly stated? | No ┈┈▶ | A well planned study has a clear hypothesis and wants to answer a specific question. Is it a question that is relevant to your situation? |

Yes ▼

| Is the sample size justified? | No ┈┈▶ | Studies which are too small can miss important effects. What size of effect could this study detect? |

Yes ▼

| Are the measurements reliable? | No ┈┈▶ | Methods of measurement should be described (and assessed for reliability) eg how do you know that subjective (or multi-centre) measurements were standardized? |

Yes ▼

| Are the statistical methods described? | No ┈┈▶ | Have they discussed their assumptions made about the data? Have they used simple analyses first before complex or multiple analyses (which may have been used to produce misleading results). |

Yes ▼

| Did the design of the study change? | Yes ▶ | Beware missing data or change in design of research during the conduct of the study, which suggest a poorly prepared study. |

No ▼

| Have the subjects been properly described? | No ┈┈▶ | How were the subjects obtained, and how do they vary (standard deviation around the mean or median) ie can the findings be generalised to your patients? |

Yes ▼

| Has statistical significance been assessed? | No ┈┈▶ | A P value below 0.05 suggests the results are unlikely to be due to chance. Confidence intervals give more information eg 3–17 mean there is a 95% chance that the true value lies within that range. |

Yes ▼

| Do you agree with the authors view about what the results mean? | No ┈┈▶ | The enthusiasm of researchers can bias their descriptions of the study and their conclusions. How do you interpret their results in the light of your own experience? Have some results not been commented on? |

Yes ▼

| Have you compared the findings to other studies? | No ┈┈▶ | New findings are usually only accepted once they are confirmed by more than one study and more than one research group. |

Yes ▼

| Should you change your management in the light of this paper? | ⇒ | If this is a high quality study, which has shown a big effect that is clinically important, with a lot of supporting evidence from previous studies, (and if it studied patients similar to yours) – the answer may be yes. |

Is the research of good quality?

Clinical decisions need to be informed and based, (as far as possible,) on information from research. We therefore need to make decisions about the quality of the research papers we read.

There are different types of research study. Controlled trials provide the most powerful type of evidence, followed by cohort studies, case-control studies and surveys. The flow chart opposite applies to all these types of research, but in addition there are some important specific questions we need to ask about each particular method, as described below:

Is it a clinical trial?

Clinical trials are used to test whether one health care intervention is superior to another. Patients with the same diagnosis are randomly allocated (double-blind, so neither the patient nor the researchers are aware of how they have been allocated) to either the new or the "current-best" treatment. The key additional questions are: Was it random allocation? Was it double-blind? Were large numbers lost to follow up and could this have biased the results?

Is it a cohort study?

Cohort studies look forward and are used to see what happens next to a group of patients. The key additional questions are: Who was eligible for the study? Was a control group used to compare results? Did follow-up occur for long enough? How was the outcome measured? Could a high drop-out rate have introduced bias?

Is it a case-control study?

Case-control studies are retrospective and used to compare a group of patients to a control group to see how they differ, in the hope that differences will bring explanations (eg the cause of an illness). The key additional questions are: Is the definition of a "case" specific enough? Is the control group appropriate? Were data collected the same way for the cases and controls?

Is it a survey?

Surveys (by questionnaires or interviews) are used to simply describe a group of individuals (eg "women with lung cancer"). It obviously has to be based on a cross-sectional sample of patients. The key additional questions are: What were the selection criteria for entry into the sample? Was the sample selected randomly from a list? Has a poor response-rate biased the results?

Is it a review paper?

Review papers combine all the results of published research (using the statistical method of meta-analysis) to detect mildly significant results. The key additional questions are: Could any important papers have been missed? How was the quality of the papers assessed? Were poor quality papers included? If so did they have a weighting to reduce their significance? Are the conclusions of the authors justified?

See also: Audit

SLEEP

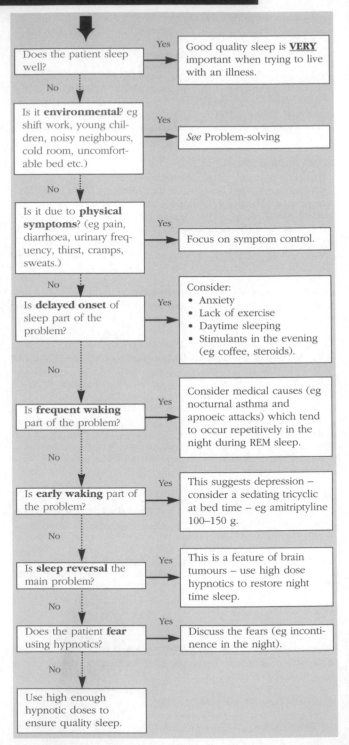

Does the patient sleep well? — Yes → Good quality sleep is **VERY** important when trying to live with an illness.

No ↓

Is it **environmental**? eg shift work, young children, noisy neighbours, cold room, uncomfortable bed etc.) — Yes → *See* Problem-solving

No ↓

Is it due to **physical symptoms**? (eg pain, diarrhoea, urinary frequency, thirst, cramps, sweats.) — Yes → Focus on symptom control.

No ↓

Is **delayed onset** of sleep part of the problem? — Yes → Consider:
- Anxiety
- Lack of exercise
- Daytime sleeping
- Stimulants in the evening (eg coffee, steroids).

No ↓

Is **frequent waking** part of the problem? — Yes → Consider medical causes (eg nocturnal asthma and apnoeic attacks) which tend to occur repetitively in the night during REM sleep.

No ↓

Is **early waking** part of the problem? — Yes → This suggests depression – consider a sedating tricyclic at bed time – eg amitriptyline 100–150 g.

No ↓

Is **sleep reversal** the main problem? — Yes → This is a feature of brain tumours – use high dose hypnotics to restore night time sleep.

No ↓

Does the patient **fear** using hypnotics? — Yes → Discuss the fears (eg incontinence in the night).

No ↓

Use high enough hypnotic doses to ensure quality sleep.

Insomnia is a very unpleasant experience that worsens most symptoms and if severe it becomes a medical emergency.

Is the patient frightened of sleeping?
Many patients feel they may die in their sleep and not wake up. This responds to explanation and establishing trust so the patient can use hypnotics. If the patients have nightmares ask about what happened and how they felt. It helps to verbalise fears and it is safer to discuss fears relating to the dream rather than to dying.

Is insomnia resistant to high dose hypnotics?
Add Chlorpromazine 25–50mg. If insomnia is severe and distressing then an IM injection of Diamorphine 2.5–5mg, Chlorpromazine 50mg Hyoscine 0.4mg guarantees 4 hours sleep for most patients.

Which hypnotic?
Temazepam (10–60mg) suits many patients, but not all. If temazepam is too powerful choose one of the very short acting hypnotics (eg zolpidem). If temazepam has little effect consider a longer active one (eg nitrazepam).

DURATION OF ACTION OF HYPNOTICS (T½)

VERY SHORT (up to 4h)	SHORT (4–12h)	INTERMEDIATE (12–20h)	LONG (>20h)
• Zolpidem (Stilnoct)	• zopiclone* (Zimovane)	• lorazepam	• nitrazepam (Mogadon)
• triazolam	• lormetazepam	• oxazepam	• flurazepam (Dalmane)
• loprazolam	• chloral (Welldorm)*		• chlordiazepoxide
	• temazepam		• diazepam

Temazepam has an active metabolic that is longer acting.

* Not benzodiazepines

What dose of hypnotic?
The dose needed is very variable but should be high enough to be effective. Sleep is very important. The dose may need to be increased after 2–3 weeks because tolerance develops to benzodiazepines if taken regularly.

SPINAL CORD COMPRESSION

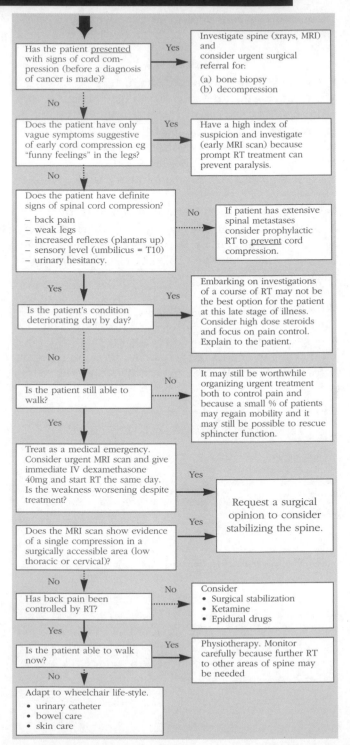

Has the patient <u>presented</u> with signs of cord compression (before a diagnosis of cancer is made)?

Yes → Investigate spine (xrays, MRI) and consider urgent surgical referral for:
(a) bone biopsy
(b) decompression

No ↓

Does the patient have only vague symptoms suggestive of early cord compression eg "funny feelings" in the legs?

Yes → Have a high index of suspicion and investigate (early MRI scan) because prompt RT treatment can prevent paralysis.

No ↓

Does the patient have definite signs of spinal cord compression?
– back pain
– weak legs
– increased reflexes (plantars up)
– sensory level (umbilicus = T10)
– urinary hesitancy.

No ····→ If patient has extensive spinal metastases consider prophylactic RT to <u>prevent</u> cord compression.

Yes ↓

Is the patient's condition deteriorating day by day?

Yes → Embarking on investigations of a course of RT may not be the best option for the patient at this late stage of illness. Consider high dose steroids and focus on pain control. Explain to the patient.

No ↓

Is the patient still able to walk?

No ····→ It may still be worthwhile organizing urgent treatment both to control pain and because a small % of patients may regain mobility and it may still be possible to rescue sphincter function.

Yes ↓

Treat as a medical emergency. Consider urgent MRI scan and give immediate IV dexamethasone 40mg and start RT the same day. Is the weakness worsening despite treatment?

Yes →

Does the MRI scan show evidence of a single compression in a surgically accessible area (low thoracic or cervical)?

Yes → Request a surgical opinion to consider stabilizing the spine.

No ↓

Has back pain been controlled by RT?

No ····→ Consider
• Surgical stabilization
• Ketamine
• Epidural drugs

Yes ↓

Is the patient able to walk now?

Yes → Physiotherapy. Monitor carefully because further RT to other areas of spine may be needed

No ↓

Adapt to wheelchair life-style.
• urinary catheter
• bowel care
• skin care

182

SPINAL CORD COMPRESSION

Is cord compression common?
10% of patients with spinal metastases develop cord compression during the course of their illness. It is usually a complication of far advanced disease, but 10–20% of these patients survive for 12 months. Cord compression may rarely occur as a presenting symptom, before the diagnosis of cancer is known.

Is this early cord compression?
The complaint of "funny feelings" in both legs should be taken very seriously, especially if there is a new thoracic spinal pain. Urgent MRI scan is indicated – even if the other signs of cord compression are not obvious. Cord compression usually occurs in the thoracic region (70)%, but may occur in the lumbosacral region (20%) or the cervical spine (10%). Lung, breast, prostate are the commonest causes.

What are the signs of cord compression?
If both legs are weak, or feel "funny" and the reflexes are brisk, and the plantar reflexes are upgoing then a cord compression is highly likely. 90% of patients will have back pain. Loss of sensation below a certain level (a "sensory level") occurs usually somewhere between nipples (T4) and the umbilicus (T10) – but may not be obvious for the first 24 hours. Urinary hesitancy is usually a late feature.

Is the patient still walking?
If the patient is still walking, emergency treatment gives a 1 in 3 chance of retaining leg strength. Act quickly – give immediate IV steroids and aim to start radiotherapy treatment within 24 hours.

Does the patient have a short prognosis?
If a patient has established cord compression and probably only has a short prognosis (eg week-by-week deterioration) it may not be in their best interests to embark on a course of radiotherapy. Discuss the options with the patient, if possible. A single treatment of radiotherapy to the spine may be adequate for pain control.

Have we set realistic short-term goals for rehabilitation?
Once the patient is paraplegic, usually with double incontinence (and impotence in men). Focus on breaking the bad news that recovery will probably not occur (rather than waiting inappropriately for strength to return). The focus of management shifts to helping the patient (and family) adjust to wheel-chair mobility and to managing the problems of paraplegia (skin and bowel care, managing a catheter, wheel-chair access to home etc). Setting realistic short-term goals is the key to good management.

SPIRITUAL DISTRESS

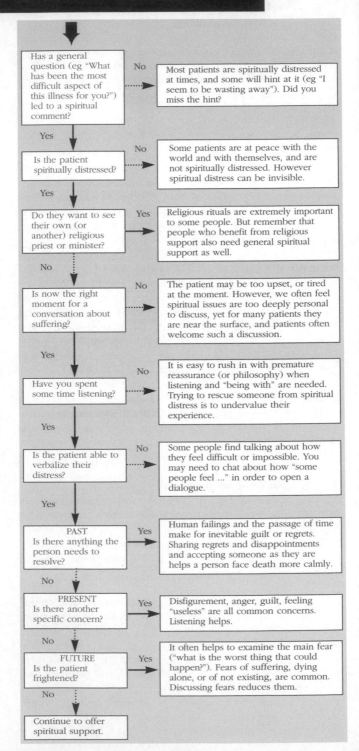

Has a general question (eg "What has been the most difficult aspect of this illness for you?") led to a spiritual comment? — **No** → Most patients are spiritually distressed at times, and some will hint at it (eg "I seem to be wasting away"). Did you miss the hint?

↓ **Yes**

Is the patient spiritually distressed? — **No** → Some patients are at peace with the world and with themselves, and are not spiritually distressed. However spiritual distress can be invisible.

↓ **Yes**

Do they want to see their own (or another) religious priest or minister? — **Yes** → Religious rituals are extremely important to some people. But remember that people who benefit from religious support also need general spiritual support as well.

↓ **No**

Is now the right moment for a conversation about suffering? — **No** → The patient may be too upset, or tired at the moment. However, we often feel spiritual issues are too deeply personal to discuss, yet for many patients they are near the surface, and patients often welcome such a discussion.

↓ **Yes**

Have you spent some time listening? — **No** → It is easy to rush in with premature reassurance (or philosophy) when listening and "being with" are needed. Trying to rescue someone from spiritual distress is to undervalue their experience.

↓ **Yes**

Is the patient able to verbalize their distress? — **No** → Some people find talking about how they feel difficult or impossible. You may need to chat about how "some people feel ..." in order to open a dialogue.

↓ **Yes**

PAST Is there anything the person needs to resolve? — **Yes** → Human failings and the passage of time make for inevitable guilt or regrets. Sharing regrets and disappointments and accepting someone as they are helps a person face death more calmly.

↓ **No**

PRESENT Is there another specific concern? — **Yes** → Disfigurement, anger, guilt, feeling "useless" are all common concerns. Listening helps.

↓ **No**

FUTURE Is the patient frightened? — **Yes** → It often helps to examine the main fear ("what is the worst thing that could happen?"). Fears of suffering, dying alone, or of not existing, are common. Discussing fears reduces them.

↓ **No**

Continue to offer spiritual support.

184

What is spiritual distress?
Medical carers often ignore the spiritual distress of their patients and yet *serious illness is often a spiritual issue* which brings a different perspective on life, a re-assessment of values and sets a person thinking about the meaning of their life.

Spiritual distress can be considered in terms of the past, present and future.

Focus	Distress	Need
PAST	• Regrets • Guilt ("It's a punishment")	• Acceptance of Self • Forgiveness
PRESENT	• Anger ("Why me") • Disgust (eg smell) • Isolation	• Sense of unity ("Why not me") • Self-esteem (eg new roles) • Social contact
FUTURE	• Fear • Pointlessness • Chaos	• Discussion about dying? • Sense of meaning • Order (eg making a will)

Is the patient mainly distressed about the past?
He or she may need to tell their life story, or to say sorry to (or re-make contact with) others or may need forgiveness for doing wrong (sometimes from a priest or minister).

Is the patient mainly distressed about the present?
He or she may need to develop a sense of belonging if they feel isolated (through companionship, feeling more in control, being accepted as themselves or finding some sense of purpose or meaning in the present situation). They may need to re-find their self-esteem, if they have lost their social roles by appreciation of their own individuality and also their own remaining responsibilities (eg to help their children).

Is the patient mainly distressed about the future?
He or she may need to discuss the practical realities of dying (which reduces unrealistic fears) or may need to sort out their affairs (making a will can be very therapeutic) or may need to develop realistic short-term goals and "appropriate hopes" (eg for the family to cope or for a future after physical death).

How can professionals help?
Professionals can relieve spiritual distress if they can offer human companionship (remembering that a good companion talks of life as well as death) and can recognize the patient as a unique person. Spiritual support is also grounded in the ordinary. Sunlight, pleasant surroundings, flowers, a comfortable chair, a pleasant smell, a view of the garden, smiles, small acts of kindness and genuine concern can all uplift the spirits.

Is formal religious support needed?
Religious support or sacraments can be a great comfort to some patients and relatives. Ask if religion is important and involve the relevant ministers or priest.

STEROIDS

Might steroids improve this symptom?	No ┈┈▶	About 40% of hospice patients benefit from a course of steroids at some point.
↓ Yes		
Have steroids already been tried for this problem?	Yes ──▶	The first course of steroids usually gives the best response for symptom control.
↓ No		
Is the patient willing to try steroids?	No ┈┈▶	Some patients are frightened of the side-effects of steroids, having seen other people have side-effects – especially weight gain or facial swelling.
↓ Yes		
Is the prognosis likely to be more than 3 months?	Yes ──▶	There is more likelihood of developing distressing side-effects (facial swelling) if steroids are used for more than a few weeks – consider postponing steroid use or consider megestrol 160mg OD as an alternative for anorexia.
↓ No		
Is the patient diabetic?	Yes ──▶	Steroids increase blood glucose. Non-insulin dependent diabetics may need to start insulin (discuss this before starting steroids) and those on insulin will probably need to increase their dose of insulin.
↓ No		
Does the patient take NSAIDS or have a history of peptic ulcer?	Yes ──▶	The risk of ulceration and perforation is increased. Give gastro-protective therapy – eg omeprazole 20mg OD.
↓ No		
Does the patient have a history of insomnia, agitation or paranoia?	Yes ──▶	Steroids can cause insomnia (therefore give early in the day) and can worsen agitation – an effective option sometimes is to give haloperidol 3–5mg daily or BD with the steroids.
↓ No		
Give a 7 day course of steroids. Has the symptom improved?	No ┈┈▶	Stop steroids if no benefit occurs. Consider other treatments.
↓ Yes		
Issue Steroid Card. Reduce dose very gradually (eg 2mg per week) to try to maintain improvement but reduce the risk of long-term steroid side-effects.	──▶	Monitor for: • oral thrush • ankle oedema • diabetes • gastric problems

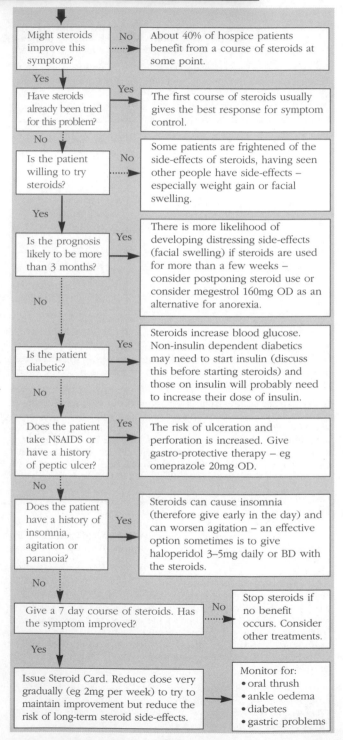

186

Who needs steroids?
50% of cancer patients benefit from steroids at some time.

What is the correct dose?
Dexamethasone is preferred because it has less mineralo-corticoid activity than prednisolone. The aim is to improve symptoms then to reduce rapidly to the lowest effective dose and to discontinue if there is no benefit.

What dose of dexamethasone?	
Dose	Indication
2 – 4 mg	Anorexia, fatigue
8 – 12 mg	To decrease tumour oedema
16 – 32 mg	Raised ICP, cord compression

Should antifungals be started?
Oral thrush is such a common complication in patients on steroids that prophylacticd Nystatin 1 ml QDS is sometimes advised routinely for <u>all</u> patients starting steroids.

Who needs gastro-protection?
About 20% of patients on steroids need gastro-protection. The risk of peptic ulceration on steroids is doubled from 1 to 2% but this means 98% are not at increased risk. Gastro-protection is indicated if a patient is on concurrent NSAID's, has had a total dose above 140 mg of Dexamethasone or has a previous history of peptic ulceration, (all of which increase the risk of ulceration or perforation). Misoprostol is the most effective treatment to protect against NSAID's otherwise ranitidine or omeprazole can be used.

How are steroids stopped?
Steroids can be stopped immediately if the patient has been on less than 6mg of Dexamethazone for less than 3 weeks (or if the patient is in the last few days of life). In other patients steroids should be stopped gradually because adrenal surpression will have occurred. The physiological dose is Dexamethasone 1 mg (Prednisolone 7 mg) so a sensible regime is to use Prednisolone 5 mg daily and reduce by 1 mg every 3 days finishing with 1 mg alternate days for a week.

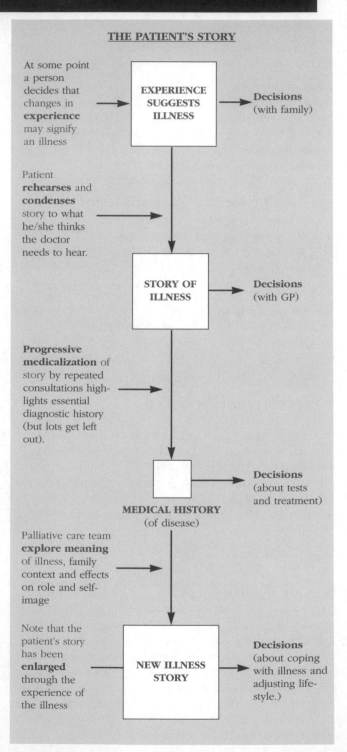

THE PATIENT'S STORY

At some point a person decides that changes in **experience** may signify an illness

EXPERIENCE SUGGESTS ILLNESS

Decisions (with family)

Patient **rehearses** and **condenses** story to what he/she thinks the doctor needs to hear.

STORY OF ILLNESS

Decisions (with GP)

Progressive medicalization of story by repeated consultations highlights essential diagnostic history (but lots get left out).

MEDICAL HISTORY (of disease)

Decisions (about tests and treatment)

Palliative care team **explore meaning** of illness, family context and effects on role and self-image

Note that the patient's story has been **enlarged** through the experience of the illness

NEW ILLNESS STORY

Decisions (about coping with illness and adjusting life-style.)

Has the patient's story become "medicalized" by repeated consultations?

A patient's story of illness gradually gets whittled down into a case history of disease. As they go through the process of diagnosis their narrative gradually shrinks to focus on the diagnostic features. Many "unremarkable" details are left out. This process is important in diagnosing disease but it means the patient tends to repeat what other doctors have found of diagnostic interest. This can lead to problems when it comes to making decisions that require an understanding of the patients individuality, emotional state and social context.

Was the patient's story rehearsed?

When patients tell their story of illness to a doctor they have usually already discussed it with several other people (family, friends or other doctors) and have usually rehearsed the story in their mind. It can be helpful to acknowledge this rehearsal process (eg "Have you been wondering how to explain all this to me") because it acknowledges the dilemma of what to tell and what to leave out and because it can enable the patient to include some important details they previously left out. It can also help in understanding the patients attitude to their illness.

Have you listened to the patient's unique story?

The way we listen to a patient's story can powerfully effect their subsequent decisions (such as whether they decide to trust you). A young women and her husband spent two hours on first meeting a hospice doctor tearfully describing their distressing encounters with doctors over the previous year (mostly small mistakes, inconsistencies of care or lack of consideration). When they had finished their story the doctor said "I would like to apologise to you on behalf of the Health Service, of which I am a part, for all the avoidable distress you have experienced over the past year". This aided their decision to comply with further therapeutic suggestions.

Have you constructed a joint narrative with the patient?

Doctors listen to the patient's story and then re-shapes the story to make medical sense and bring some order out of chaos. Patients emerge from an encounter with a doctor bearing a new story about the nature and significance of their illness. When the new narrative is jointly constructed (which involves shared decision-making) it gives some power back to the patient and makes it much more likely that the patient will comply with suggested treatments. It is also an important ethical safeguard within the doctor-patient relationship.

A lot of decision-making happens through stories

Most *patients* relate to stories better than they relate to statistics or probabilities. For example, if a doctor says to a patient "I had another patient the same age as you with the same condition who had this operation a month ago and she has done really well, and is very glad she had it done" it can be very persuasive, but obviously should not replace a factual explanation of risks and benefits.

See Also: Consultations

SUBCUTANEOUS DRUGS

WHICH DRUGS FOR SC INFUSION?

DRUG AMPOULES	STARTING DOSE PER 24 HOUR	MAIN USE	NOTES
Diamorphine 10,30,100,500 mg	15 mg	Pain	These drugs are often mixed together in combinations of 2, 3 (and sometimes 4) with good effect. This is established good practice but outside the licensing indications for most of the drugs.

Definitive data on their compatibilities is still lacking. Seek advice if unsure which drugs to use. |
Cyclizine 50 mg/1 ml	100 mg	Sickness	
Metoclopramide 10 mg/2 ml	30 mg	Sickness	
Haloperidol 5 mg/1 ml	2.5 mg	Drug-induced nausea	
Methotrimeprazine 25 mg/1 ml	12.5 mg	Broad-spectrum powerful anti-emetic	
Midazolam 10 mg/2 ml	10 mg	Agitation Anti-convulsant	
Hyoscine hydrobromide 0.4 mg/1 ml 0.6 mg/1 ml	1.2 mg	Bubbling	
Buscopan (hyoscine butylbromide) 20 mg/1 ml	40 mg	Colic	
Dexamethasone 4 mg/1 ml	4 mg	Reduces peri tumour oedema	Add last & slowly. Does not mix with cylizine
Octreotide 100 mcg/1 ml 500 mcg/1 ml	100 mcg	Reduces gastro-intestinal secretions	Does not mix with cyclizine or dexamethasone
Ketamine 500 mg/5 ml	100 mg	Difficult pain problems	Strong non-opioid. Mixes with diamorphine, haloperidol or midazolam. Dose range 100–600 mg per 24 hour.
Phenobarbitone 200 mg/1 ml	200 mg	Anti-convulsant	Use separate pump
Diclofenac 75 mg/3 ml	150 mg	Severe bone pain	• Use separate pump

• Avoid in renal failure |
| **Ondansetron** 2 mg/1 ml | 8 mg | Chemotherapy induced nausea | Use separate pump. |
| **Hyaluronidase** 1500 units/ ampoule | 1500 units | Dispersal of SC fluids. (May also decrease inflammation at injection site | Prime the line with it. Not if allergy or asthma. |

Which drugs can be given subcutaneously?

Many drugs are effective via a subcutaneous infusion. Common combinations include diamorphine, cyclizine and Buscopan (eg in malignant intestinal obstruction) or diamorhine, midazolam and hyoscine (eg in the terminal phase). The number of drugs being given by the SC route is steadily increasing with experience.

Which drugs can be combined?

Which drugs are combined is based on clinical experience of what works. Many drugs will mix together without precipitation and are clinically effective (although it remains unknown whether partial inactivation is occurring). Drugs which tend to precipitate with other drugs are cyclizine and dexamethasone – if precipitation in a mixture is occurring it is often due to one of these drugs. Certain drugs need to be given in a separate syringe pump, eg diclofenac, phenobarbitone.

Are the drugs licensed for this use?

In Palliative Medicine about 15% of prescriptions are for unlicensed indications.

Many drugs given by the SC route are not licensed for use in this way. The Medicines Act of 1968 permit the use of unlicensed medicines, or licensed drugs for unlicensed purposes provided the prescriber is acting in concordance with past practice of others in the field. Legally the doctor must be aware of the licence status of the drug and as with all prescribing, should use reasonable skill and care, and normally have the patient's informed consent – eg it should have been explained carefully first.

What if a skin reaction occurs?

Skin reactions can occur especially with cyclizine and methotrimeprazine and the site then needs changing daily. Increasing the dilution (use a 30cc syringe) can help. Some patients are allergic to the metal in the butterfly – use a plastic cannula. Non–sterile technique can result in abscesses.

See also: Subcutaneous infusions

SUBCUTANEOUS INFUSION

Is there an **indication** for SC infusion?
- persistent nausea?
or
- difficulty swallowing?
or
- malabsorbtion?

No → <u>Oral</u> analgesia is just as effective as by SC infusion

Yes ↓

Are there any contra-indications?

Yes → Use alternative route if:
- Platelets are below 10×10^9/L (it may cause bleeding).
- Bullous skin disorders.

Yes ↓

Is the necessary **equipment** available?

No →
- Syringe driver (Graseby MS26 is best)
- Butterfly with long tubing
- Drugs and prescription for repeats
- Water for injection
- Holster (or 'bum bag')
- Trained staff

Yes ↓

Has the patient been involved in the **decision**?

No → The patient may fear a gadget, or believe a pump is associated with dying. Listen to concerns and explain.

Yes ↓

Do you know which **drugs** to use?

No → A common starting combination is diamorphine with cyclizine. See Subcutaneous Drugs.

Yes ↓

Do you know what **dose of diamorphine** should be added?

No → Use 50% of oral morphine dose – eg if patient is pain free on MST 90 mg BD put 90 mg diamorphine per 24h in the pump.

Yes ↓

Have you explained the system to the patient and carers?

No →
- May need initial IM injection
- Under skin (not in a vein)
- Safe and simple
- Refilled once a day
- Site changed every 2–3 days
- Pump not water-proof
- Light flashes every 25 seconds (no flash = low battery = still runs for 24 hours)
- New battery lasts 50 days
- 10 second warning beep = blocked
- Beeps every 0.23 mm
- Check 6 hourly for
  - correct volume remaining
  - light flashing
  - no leaks

Yes ↓

Have the drugs **crystallized**?

Yes →
- Discard mixture, syringe and line
- Increase dilution (consider 30 ml syringe)
- Change cyclizine to alternative anti-emetic
- Use 2 pumps and/or consult pharmacist
- If it happened while in use, re-site needle
- Keep away from sunlight or heat

No ↓

Have I discussed future **plans**?

No →
- How long can it stay in?
- What if it dosen't work?
- Oral medication can still be taken once nausea settles

Yes ↓

Follow-up

↓

Has **irritation** developed at the injection site?

Yes →
- Change site
- Change irritant drugs (cyclizine or methotrimeprazine)
- Increase dilution
- Try plastic cannula (eg Abbocath 26g)

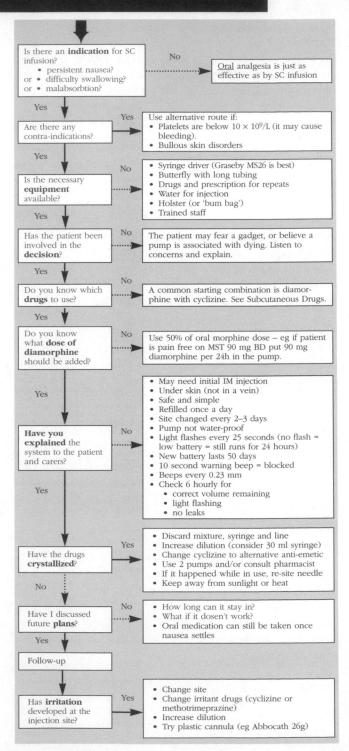

192

SUBCUTANEOUS INFUSION

When is a syringe driver indicated?

A syringe driver is used to provide a subcutaneous infusion of drugs and is indicated if oral medication cannot be taken because of vomiting or dysphagia or weakness in the terminal stages (or rarely malabsorbtion).

What is involved?

A butterfly needle is sited subcutaneously (usually in the upper chest or abdomen, occasionally on the upper arm or back). The butterfly has a long tube and is connected to a syringe driver, a small light weight device that the patient carries either in a holster or a "bumbag" (or bedbound patients tuck them under the pillow). Once the needle is in place it may last several days, although some patients get redness and soreness due to some of the drugs (particularly cyclizine and methotrimeprazine) and it sometimes needs to be change daily. The syringe driver is refilled every 24 hours, which can be done by the district nurse at home.

Is it permanent?

It can be used long-term. Some patients have it for many months (eg for dyphagia). More commonly it is used for 1–2 weeks to control nausea and vomiting and then the patient is gradually weaned back onto oral medication.

How is it stopped?

Usually it is best to start the patient on oral antimetics and gradually reduce the dose of antimetics in the infusion. If the nausea and vomiting remain well-controlled the patient can then transferred onto the equivalent dose of analgesic orally and the infusion can be stopped (eg if the patient is having diamorphine 100mg per 24 hours via the pump and is pain controlled they will need MST 100mg BD orally).

What is the correct dose of SC diamorphine?

The equi-analgesic conversion ratio of oral morphine to SC diamorphine is somewhere between 1 : 2 and 1 : 3. Personally I use 1 : 2 because it is simple and effective, as an initial step. The dose may need slight daily adjustment up or down.

See also: Subcutaneous drugs

SUPPORT

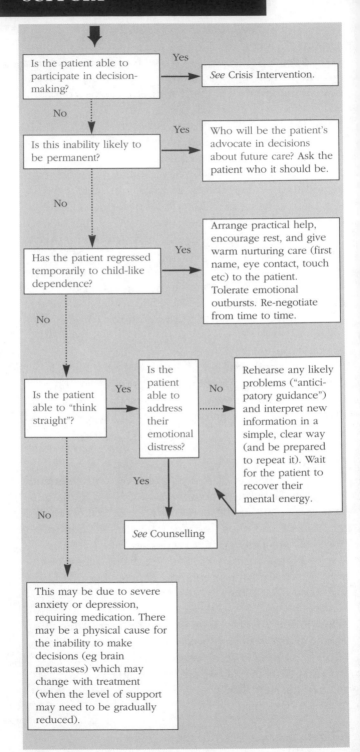

Is the patient able to participate in decision-making?

Yes → *See* Crisis Intervention.

No

Is this inability likely to be permanent?

Yes → Who will be the patient's advocate in decisions about future care? Ask the patient who it should be.

No

Has the patient regressed temporarily to child-like dependence?

Yes → Arrange practical help, encourage rest, and give warm nurturing care (first name, eye contact, touch etc) to the patient. Tolerate emotional outbursts. Re-negotiate from time to time.

No

Is the patient able to "think straight"?

Yes → Is the patient able to address their emotional distress?

No → Rehearse any likely problems ("anticipatory guidance") and interpret new information in a simple, clear way (and be prepared to repeat it). Wait for the patient to recover their mental energy.

Yes → *See* Counselling

No → This may be due to severe anxiety or depression, requiring medication. There may be a physical cause for the inability to make decisions (eg brain metastases) which may change with treatment (when the level of support may need to be gradually reduced).

194

What is support?
Support is a style of care appropriate to patients who are having difficulty participating in decision-making. It involves warm nurturing care, arranging practical help, interpreting new information, rehearsing problems with the patient, optimism, tolerating abnormal behaviour, mediating between family members and encouraging rest.

When is support needed?
The patient needs support if they are too exhausted emotionally or mentally to take part in decision-making about their own care.

Is the patient too emotionally distressed to "think straight"?
Emotional distress may block decision-making. It may be short-term distress (part of an adjustment reaction) and only last a few days. Or the distress may be a more profound emotional reaction (possibly relating to childhood experiences) that needs some formal counselling sessions.

Has the patient 'regressed'?
A personality-shift of regression to a more child-like state is common for a time in patients with physical illness (although occasionally it can be permanent). Regression often subsides after a time of rest and support when the patient can be gently challenged by professionals to re-adopt the "adult" ego state (moving from a "parent-child" back to an "adult-adult" pattern of interaction – see Transactional Analysis).

How does support relate to other styles of care?
The four key roles of professionals are: Explanation, Support, Problem solving and Counselling.
  Most patients need all these approaches at different times. Many factors will effect decisions about which style of care is appropriate (especially the patient's personality and the stage of the illness. This idea is discussed further in the section of Crisis Intervention.

How much support is needed?
The support needed gradually reduces as the crisis resolves and the patient begins to adjust and re-finds energy for problem solving (see diagram below).

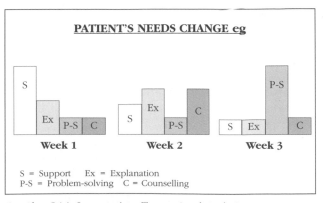

PATIENT'S NEEDS CHANGE eg

Week 1   Week 2   Week 3

S = Support   Ex = Explanation
P-S = Problem-solving   C = Counselling

See Also: Crisis Intervention, Transactional Analysis.

TERMINAL PHASE

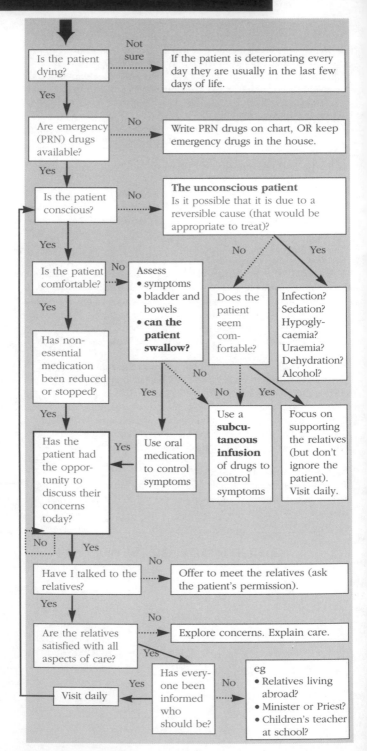

Is the patient dying? — **Not sure** → If the patient is deteriorating every day they are usually in the last few days of life.

Yes ↓

Are emergency (PRN) drugs available? — **No** → Write PRN drugs on chart, OR keep emergency drugs in the house.

Yes ↓

Is the patient conscious? — **No** → **The unconscious patient**
Is it possible that it is due to a reversible cause (that would be appropriate to treat)?

No ↙   **Yes** ↘

Yes ↓

Is the patient comfortable? — **No** → Assess
• symptoms
• bladder and bowels
• **can the patient swallow?**

Does the patient seem comfortable?

Infection?
Sedation?
Hypoglycaemia?
Uraemia?
Dehydration?
Alcohol?

Yes ↓

Has non-essential medication been reduced or stopped?

No → Use a **subcutaneous infusion** of drugs to control symptoms

Yes → Focus on supporting the relatives (but don't ignore the patient). Visit daily.

Yes ↓

Use oral medication to control symptoms

Has the patient had the opportunity to discuss their concerns today? — **Yes** ↑

No →

Yes ↓

Have I talked to the relatives? — **No** → Offer to meet the relatives (ask the patient's permission).

Yes ↓

Are the relatives satisfied with all aspects of care? — **No** → Explore concerns. Explain care.

Yes ↓

Has everyone been informed who should be? — **No** → eg
• Relatives living abroad?
• Minister or Priest?
• Children's teacher at school?

Yes → Visit daily

196

Is the patient dying?

The diagnosis of "dying" is VERY important because it changes medical decision-making. Once a patient is diagnosed as dying:

- investigations become irrelevant
- aiming to prolong life becomes irrelevant
- patient comfort takes priority
- increased support for the family is needed

If the patient has a progressive incurable disease, if reversible causes of deterioration have been excluded (eg infection hypercalcaemia) and if they are very weak and drowsy and getting weaker every day, then they are dying.

What is the role of the doctor?

The doctor continues to have a key role when a patient is dying (and some doctors seem to be unaware of this):

- visit daily
- liaise with nursing team
- asses patient's comfort
- review medication
- support the relatives (see Family Meetings)

Families are always very grateful for the skilled medical supervision of their dying relative.

How do I monitor an unconscious patient?

Visit daily, liaise with the nursing team about nursing care (eye care, mouth care regular timing, catheter care, bowel care). Monitor medication and assess level of consciousness, using EYELID FLICKER TEST. When the eyelid is touched in deeply unconscious patients there is no effect. Relatives find it reassuring when the doctor talks to a patient even when unconscious (eg "It is Dr Kaye, Michael, I am just going to touch your eyelid and test a reflex".)

What medication is used?

A subcutaneous infusion of drugs is very helpful if the patients can no longer swallow. A common combination is diamorphine (for pain or dyspnoea), hyoscine (to dry up respiratory secretions and control the terminal bubbling) and midazolam if there is any terminal agitation.

- Diamorphine   mg\24hr (dose = 50% oral morphine\24hr)
- Hyoscine   0.8–1.6 mg\24hr
- Midazolam   10–60 mg\24hr

How can the patient be protected from too many visitors?

Many dying patients have a dilemma about visitors, wanting the support but getting exhausted by TOO MANY (well meaning) VISITORS – consider a "medical edict" to set limits and suggest a visiting rota (so visitors can also get some rest).

See also Dehydration, Dying, Family Meetings, Subcutaneous Infusions.

THINKING

Is the patient able to think?
Medical decision-making is a foreign country to many patients, who can feel overwhelmed by their situation. Even simple medical decisions may feel confusing if the patient has a rigid personality (eg low toleration of risk, rigid holding onto dogma), difficulty thinking (confusion/depression/dementia/brain tumour), low IQ or low assertiveness.

How do we think?
The brain works by pattern recognition. To save us having to make too many decisions we form habits of thinking and acting. This has 2 important advantages: If we recognise one part of a pattern we can rapidly call up the whole pattern – enhancing recognition. Secondly it allows us form time-saving sequences of behaviour. For example, we have a routine for getting dressed so we don't have to waste mental energy deciding on the best order for putting on our clothes (there are theoretically 39 million possible ways of putting on 11 articles of clothing!).

Is your own thinking too rigid?
But pattern-recognition tends to make us think in stereotypes, so that we see only what we are prepared to see. If a situation triggers an already known problem, it can save time, but it can make us lazy about the decision-making process. When we say "this patient reminds me of" we begin to recall patterns and to assume the situation is not new.

   When we are very familiar with the "medical route" we can forget what is involved in making "simple" decisions, and fail to see the patient's perspective (see box opposite).

Has logic been applied?
We often have to take information and then draw a logical conclusion from it. The difficulty is that two premises may be true but the conclusion drawn from them can still be false. This is discussed in more detail in the Introduction.

Have you given the patient enough time to think?
See box below.

Imagine a road -block

Consider the route you take to work every morning. It becomes "second nature" and you can get to work without thinking about it.

But imagine that one day there is a road block right outside your own home and instead of turning left you have to go right (or vice versa). You will need to spend some time making decisions about which way to go – you may even need to consult a map. When you get to work you will want to share your feelings of frustration (ie there is an emotional element to decision-making). **Familiarity with a route leads us to forget all the difficulties of the original decision-making process**. Similarly, what seems obvious to us, as specialists, is often not obvious to patients at all. We forget how much time is needed to think, analyse and reflect in any unfamiliar situation. This is why simply stating the obvious can be surprisingly helpful when giving explanations to patients and families.

Have you considered thinking aloud?
A study in the Netherlands of how GP's registrars made decisions, found that thinking aloud gave better insight into their decision-making process than retrospective verbal reports. Thinking aloud led to more reflection on alternative options, and the various aspects of each treatment. They found that common decisions were often made too routinely, with little reflection about alternative options. They concluded that thinking aloud is a good method of teaching and learning more about medical decision-making, but that it could not be used during an actual patient consultation. But I wonder. Thinking aloud about the rationale behind a medical decision and the limits of treatment may increase a patient's understanding of the decision, which could be very helpful for many patients.

See also Consultations, Decision-making.

TISSUE DONATION

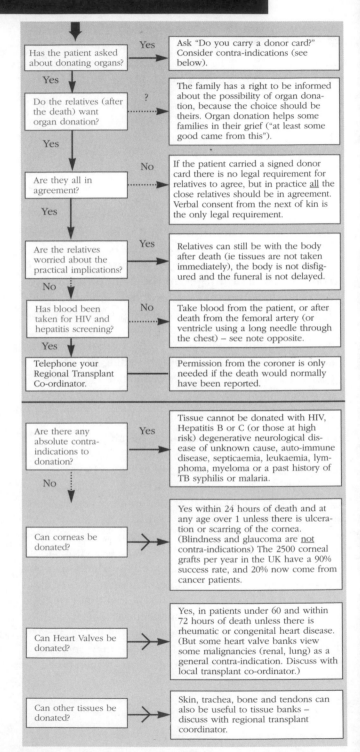

Has the patient asked about donating organs?	**Yes** →	Ask "Do you carry a donor card?" Consider contra-indications (see below).
Yes ↓		
Do the relatives (after the death) want organ donation?	**?** ⋯→	The family has a right to be informed about the possibility of organ donation, because the choice should be theirs. Organ donation helps some families in their grief ("at least some good came from this").
Yes ↓		
Are they all in agreement?	**No** ⋯→	If the patient carried a signed donor card there is no legal requirement for relatives to agree, but in practice all the close relatives should be in agreement. Verbal consent from the next of kin is the only legal requirement.
Yes ↓		
Are the relatives worried about the practical implications?	**Yes** →	Relatives can still be with the body after death (ie tissues are not taken immediately), the body is not disfigured and the funeral is not delayed.
No ↓		
Has blood been taken for HIV and hepatitis screening?	**No** ⋯→	Take blood from the patient, or after death from the femoral artery (or ventricle using a long needle through the chest) – see note opposite.
Yes ↓		
Telephone your Regional Transplant Co-ordinator.	→	Permission from the coroner is only needed if the death would normally have been reported.

Are there any absolute contra-indications to donation?	**Yes** →	Tissue cannot be donated with HIV, Hepatitis B or C (or those at high risk) degenerative neurological disease of unknown cause, auto-immune disease, septicaemia, leukaemia, lymphoma, myeloma or a past history of TB syphilis or malaria.
No ↓		
Can corneas be donated?	→	Yes within 24 hours of death and at any age over 1 unless there is ulceration or scarring of the cornea. (Blindness and glaucoma are _not_ contra-indications) The 2500 corneal grafts per year in the UK have a 90% success rate, and 20% now come from cancer patients.
Can Heart Valves be donated?	→	Yes, in patients under 60 and within 72 hours of death unless there is rheumatic or congenital heart disease. (But some heart valve banks view some malignancies (renal, lung) as a general contra-indication. Discuss with local transplant co-ordinator.)
Can other tissues be donated?	→	Skin, trachea, bone and tendons can also be useful to tissue banks – discuss with regional transplant coordinator.

Can patients with cancer donate organs?

Malignancy is generally a contra-indication to organ donation (heart, lung, kidneys, bowel, pancreas, liver) but tissues CAN still be donated (corneas, heart valves, skin, bone, tendons, trachea).

Does the patient carry a donor card?

30% of the population of the UK carry donor cards. However at least half of these patients are overlooked because of the perceived difficulty in discussing the situation with the patient or the family.

What is the maximum time from death to organ removal?

Vital organs suffer irreversible ischaemic damage following asystole but corneas, heart valves and other tissues remain viable for transplant purposes for a limited time. Corneas remain viable for 24 hours, heart valve for 72 hours.

What are the legal requirements?

Written consent for organ donation is not necessary in the UK. Verbal consent from the next-of-kin is the only requirement.

Are blood tests needed?

A 20ml clotted blood sample is essential (to test for hepatitis B and C, HIV and syphilis). They can be taken before or immediately after death.

Does the Coroner need to be informed?

Permission is only needed from the coroner if a death is related to industrial disease or it is normally one that needs to be reported to the coroner.

Is there a protocol?

It is very helpful to have an in-house protocol for tissue donation so that staff know what to do when patients or relatives ask about it. A poster about tissue donation in the coffee area can encourage enquiries. Your local Regional Transplant Co-ordinator can advise you on setting up an educational session for staff.

TRANSACTIONAL ANALYSIS

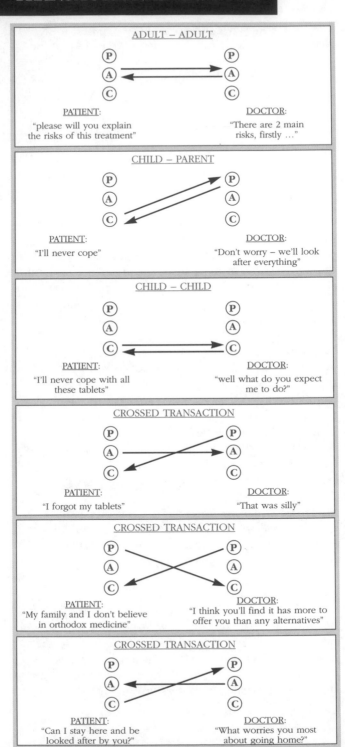

ADULT – ADULT

(P)   (P)
(A) ⟷ (A)
(C)   (C)

PATIENT:
"please will you explain the risks of this treatment"

DOCTOR:
"There are 2 main risks, firstly …"

CHILD – PARENT

PATIENT:
"I'll never cope"

DOCTOR:
"Don't worry – we'll look after everything"

CHILD – CHILD

PATIENT:
"I'll never cope with all these tablets"

DOCTOR:
"well what do you expect me to do?"

CROSSED TRANSACTION

PATIENT:
"I forgot my tablets"

DOCTOR:
"That was silly"

CROSSED TRANSACTION

PATIENT:
"My family and I don't believe in orthodox medicine"

DOCTOR:
"I think you'll find it has more to offer you than any alternatives"

CROSSED TRANSACTION

PATIENT:
"Can I stay here and be looked after by you?"

DOCTOR:
"What worries you most about going home?"

Parallel Transactions

Transactional analysis is a very useful framework for understanding some of the barriers to decision making. It is a model that assesses which "ego state" each person is using during the transaction, "Parent", "Adult" or "Child". There is often more than one type of transaction during a conversation.

ADULT – ADULT transactions are generally the most useful for shared decision-making with patients. But decision-making is often complicated by other types of transaction.

CHILD – PARENT transactions are common, because ill people often regress to a child-like state at times of intense stress. This is a style of interaction that can be appropriate when providing support to the patient (*see* Support). The nurturing "Parent" part of the carer responds to the vulnerable "Child" part of the patient. It is a parallel transaction which in theory can go on forever. At some point however it is often challenged by an Adult – Adult response from the carer (see last box, below).

CHILD – CHILD transactions are occasionally appropriate when relating to patients at the human level (eg swapping spontaneous stories or jokes) but are usually inappropriate and unhelpful when trying to get on with the "Adult" task of decision-making. If the doctor's CHILD is responding due to tiredness or emotional immaturity it is especially unhelpful. Either the doctor or patient will have to change the situation by making an ADULT – ADULT comment.

Crossed Transactions

Crossed Transactions (ie not parallel) tend to bring the conversation to a halt, until another (parallel) transaction is negotiated.

PARENT–CHILD transactions that feel critical can block shared decision-making. A "parental" approach to patients can be appropriate to the relationship at times (if it is affirming or helping to set boundaries)

PARENT – CHILD crossed transactions can turn into a battle unless the transaction is manoeuvred round to an ADULT – ADULT transaction. If the patient maintains the 'PARENT' state, the doctor may need to step down to "CHILD", to make the transaction parallel and move the conversation forward (eg "I am feeling confused – what do you think is the way forward?")

CHILD – PARENT transactions may need to be challenged at the appropriate time by and ADULT – ADULT response from the professional. A patient who is frightened and regressed may be unable to participate in decision-making. That situation may be maintained if a professional always responds as a nurturing "Parent". But initiating an ADULT – ADULT transaction may allow the patient to start sharing in decisions again.

See also: Support.

WEAKNESS

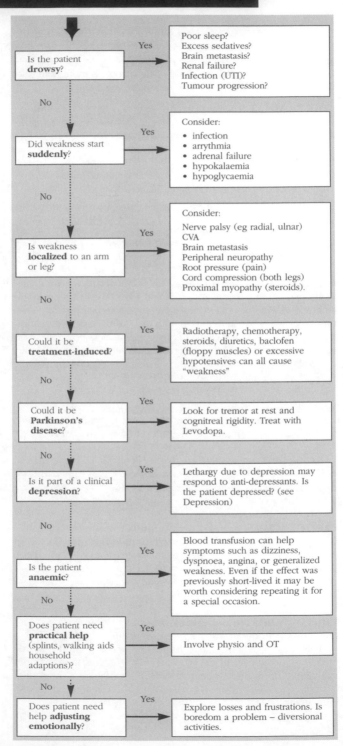

Is the patient drowsy? — Yes →
Poor sleep?
Excess sedatives?
Brain metastasis?
Renal failure?
Infection (UTI)?
Tumour progression?

No ↓

Did weakness start suddenly? — Yes →
Consider:
- infection
- arrythmia
- adrenal failure
- hypokalaemia
- hypoglycaemia

No ↓

Is weakness localized to an arm or leg? — Yes →
Consider:
Nerve palsy (eg radial, ulnar)
CVA
Brain metastasis
Peripheral neuropathy
Root pressure (pain)
Cord compression (both legs)
Proximal myopathy (steroids).

No ↓

Could it be treatment-induced? — Yes →
Radiotherapy, chemotherapy, steroids, diuretics, baclofen (floppy muscles) or excessive hypotensives can all cause "weakness"

No ↓

Could it be Parkinson's disease? — Yes →
Look for tremor at rest and cognitreal rigidity. Treat with Levodopa.

No ↓

Is it part of a clinical depression? — Yes →
Lethargy due to depression may respond to anti-depressants. Is the patient depressed? (see Depression)

No ↓

Is the patient anaemic? — Yes →
Blood transfusion can help symptoms such as dizziness, dyspnoea, angina, or generalized weakness. Even if the effect was previously short-lived it may be worth considering repeating it for a special occasion.

No ↓

Does patient need practical help (splints, walking aids household adaptions)? — Yes →
Involve physio and OT

No ↓

Does patient need help adjusting emotionally? — Yes →
Explore losses and frustrations. Is boredom a problem – diversional activities.

What does "weak" mean?

Does the patient mean muscular weakness, drowsiness, frailty and unsteadiness (are they having falls?) or do they mean cowardly or frightened.

What is the main problem?

Explore the problem. Has impairment (weak legs) led do some disability (eg difficulty being mobile) or some social handicap (eg "can't get to the shops") or emotional/spiritual distress ("I'm fading away" "I'm dying").

Is the weakness generalised?

Almost all patients with progressive illness experience generalised weakness. Loss of general strength seems to correlate with a shortening prognosis. However sometimes the weakness is localised due to a neurological problem in the brain, spinal cord, nerve or muscle, which may be reversible with treatment.

Is there a reversible cause?

Weakness of progressive diseases usually has a very gradual onset. If the weakness is of sudden onset exclude an under-lying medical complication. Consider blood tests, MSU, chest Xray and ECG.

Is it part of depression?

Depression can be overlooked but greatly worsens lethargy or weakness and may respond to antidepressants.

Is the patient anaemic?

Anaemia is usually normocytic. If Hb is below 8g/dl, symptoms can be improved by a blood transfusion. Has the patient had a blood transfusion previously? Did it help and for how long?. A trial of blood transfusion is always worthwhile if the patient is anaemic, especially if transfusion has been helpful in the past.

Has physiotherapy or OT been considered?

Maximising remaining strength improves morale and self-esteem. OT can help with practical adaptions in the home and social adjustment to life-style and role.

Does the patient need emotional help?

The most difficult part of progressive illness for most patients is adjusting to weakness and loss of independence and facing the frustration of not being able to do things that they previously enjoyed. Adjusting can involve changes in social role and changes in activity. The patient often benefits from some specific counselling to help them make the adjustment (both practical and emotional). (*See* Counselling).

The internet has been around for approximately 30 years, originally for information exchange between computers in government and university institutions.

The World Wide Web began in 1992. Up till then the Internet was used mainly by academics and the military, but it suddenly became accessible to everyone after a British scientist called Tim Berners-Lee, working in Geneva invented hypertext. This uses linked references to track down text on databases around the world. Hypertext soon became the standard way of transferring documents around the internet, and the World Wide Web (WWW) was born, bringing the world's knowledge base to our desktops. By 1996 the web had 40 million users worldwide. Berners-Lee missed out on worldwide fame because he did not patent his idea, but optimistically pointed out, "at least I'm not chased by photographers every day".

The World Wide Web is a useful way of getting information from the Internet. It is a collection of files containing text and graphics (and sound and video) which can be viewed on any computer connected to the internet using a "web browser" program (eg Netscape Navigator). Files are accessed by typing in their unique resource location (URL) address. Pages are interconnected so that references to other pages on the same computer or elsewhere can be obtained using hyper-text links.

The benefit of the Internet for the medical profession is the rapid accessibility of a vast amount of information. Unfortunately medical information from reputable sources can be indistinguishable from that provided by less reliable agents, but, used in an organised manner, the information can be more accurate and up to date than that provided in any other way.

If you do not know the address, or wish to find new sites, the WWW allows a page to be found by typing keywords into a specialized database called a search engine (eg Alta Vista) but these can provide a large amount of irrelevant material. Fortunately, there are now several high quality medical search services such as Medical Matrix (**www.medmatrix.org/index.asp**), OMNI (**www.omni.ac.uk**) and CliniWeb (**www.ohsu. edu/cliniweb**).

Medline is an extremely useful resource but there is a delay of some weeks before papers are entered onto the database. Grateful Med (**www.igm.nlm.nig.gov/**) is a free Medline and Medline search filters will improve search results (**www.ihs.ox.ac.uk/library/filters.html**). Note that

Medline search is not the same as an Internet search. WebMedLit (**www.webmedlit.com**) is a database covering 23 mainstream medical journals. It updates nightly by scanning the web for new articles.

Discussion groups of interested parties can exchange information and can send newsletters via email to all subscribers.

SOME USEFUL SITES

- Medical internet search
  www.mwsearch.com/

- Cochrane Database
  hiru.mcmaster.ca/COCHRANE/DEFAULT.HTM

- Oncolink Multimedia Oncology
  Cancer.med.upenn.edu.

- Doctors Guide to the Internet
  www.pslgroup.com/DOCGUIDE.HTM

- European Journal of Palliative Care
  www.ejpc.co.uk/

- Progress in Palliative Care
  www.leeds.ac.uk/lmi/ppc/ppcmain.html

- Palliative Medicine Journal
  www.healthworks.co.uk/hw/publisher/arnold/arnold4.html

Some search strategies

neuropathic pain	will find web pages containing the words "neuropathic" and/or "pain".
neuropathic-pain	will find web pages containing the term "neuropathic pain" rather than all web pages containing either word in isolation.
neuropathic or neuropathy	will find web pages containing the word "neuropathic" and/or "neuropathy".
pain NEAR neuropathic	will list web pages where the words "pain" and "neuropathic" appear near to each other in the text.
pain AND NOT neuropathic	will list web pages where the word "pain" appears but the word "neuropathic" does not.

For information on search strategies, visit
http://www.altavista.com/av/content/help_advanced.htm

What is the Cochrane Collaboration?

The Cochrane collaboration is a network of experts undertaking regular reviews of randomised controlled trials in health care. The UK Cochrane Centre (UKCC) was established first as part of the NHS Research and Development Programme in October 1992, and led to an international network of individuals and institutions, with Cochrane Centres now in some 12 countries.

The task of the Cochrane Collaboration is to prepare, maintain, and disseminate systematic, up-to-date reviews of RCT's of health care, and, when RCTs are not available, reviews of the most reliable evidence from other sources.

The Cochrane centres are not directly responsible for preparing and maintaining systematic reviews. This is the responsibility of collaborative review groups (which also maintain registers of reviews). Cochrane reviews are not subject to copyright. The Cochrane Collaboration thus belongs to all the contributors, collectively.

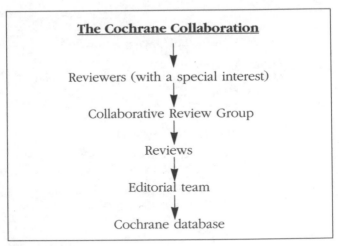

The Cochrane Collaboration

↓

Reviewers (with a special interest)

↓

Collaborative Review Group

↓

Reviews

↓

Editorial team

↓

Cochrane database

The aim is to establish review groups to cover the whole of medicine. There are currently over 50 review groups. About 20 have their editorial bases in the UK (although all have strong links with organisations abroad especially in the USA, Australia and Japan.)

A review group may have 20-100 reviewers responsible for writing new systematic reviews of RCTs and updating previous reviews of RCTs (updated quarterly). All the Cochrane groups depend on enthusiasm and collaboration.

Reviews have to be scientific

Review articles need to constructed in a scientific way, with clearly specified methods of identifying, selecting and validating the information that is included, otherwise readers may end up with false conclusions. Has the available evidence been selected in an unbiased way? Is there enough consistency in the trials to warrant pooling the results? Are the pooled results statistically valid?

How did it start?

In 1972 Archie Cochrane wrote an influential book, *Effectiveness and Efficiency: Random Reflections on Health Services*. He suggested that, because resources are limited, they should be used to provide effective health care. He drew attention to the collective ignorance about the effects of health care, and explained how evidence from randomised controlled trials (RCT's) could help us to use resources more rationally. In 1979, he wrote; "It is surely a great criticism of our profession that we have not organised a critical summary, by speciality or subspecialty adapted periodically, of all relevant randomised controlled trials." Cochrane's simple ideas were soon widely recognised and supported, but progress in applying his principles has been very slow because the valid evidence is not readily accessible when making decisions.

The Cochrane Library

The Cochrane Library.is a quarterly publication (on CD-Rom and the Internet) containing 4 databases.

Databases in the Cochrane library

- Cochrane database of Systematic Reviews (CDSR)
- Cochrane Controlled trials register (CCTR)
- Database of Abstracts of Reviews of Effectiveness (DARE)
- Review Methodology (research methods used to write reviews).
- Reviewer's handbook (jargon, contacts for review groups)

Cochrane library

- **http://hiru.mcmaster.ca/cochrane/default.htm** or **www.cochrane.co.uk**

Palliative Care and Cochrane

The Pain, Palliative and Support Care Group (PaPaS) started in January 1998. So far there are reviews on:

- Anti-convulsants for acute and chronic pain:
- Radiotherapy for bony metastases
- Acute Pain Treatments

There are also protocols (forerunners to full reviews) on:

- Acupuncture for chronic headache
- Steroids for malignant bowel obstruction.
- Cachexia

The PaPaS website

The PaPaS group is keen to recruit reviewers and searchers. For information on involvement contact:

Mrs F Fairman
Review Group Co-ordinator
Pain Research Unit
Churchill Hospital
Oxford OX3 7LJ

Or via the website http://www.jr2.ox.ac.uk/Cochrane

The Cochrane Logo

The Cochrane Collaboration logo represents a systematic review of data from seven RCT's (on steroids in premature labour to prevent respiratory distress in premature babies). Each horizontal line represents the results of one trial (the shorter the line, the more certain the result). If a horizontal line touches the vertical line, it means there was no clear difference between the treatments. The *diamond* to the left of the vertical line represents the combined results of the 7 trials and indicates that the treatment is beneficial (and reduces the death rate by 30-50%). These 7 trials were published by 1982, but it was only after 1989 when a systematic review of all the RCTs was published that most doctors began to realize it was an effective treatment.

The Cochrane logo

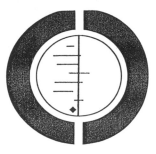

Who was Archie Cochrane?

A L Cochrane was a Scottish physician who qualified in medicine in 1948 at UCH in London. During the war he was captured and spent 5 years as a medical officer to prisoners of war. After the war he spent 10 years at the MRC's pneumoconiosis research unit and then became professor of chest diseases at the Welsh National School of Medicine, before finally becoming Director of the MRC's epidemiology unit in Cardiff. His 1971 book "Effectiveness and Efficiency: random reflections on health services" had a widespread international effect. Although he emphasised the importance of randomized controlled trials he was very aware that decisions about patient care are complex, and that undue emphasis on "evidence" may sometimes be inappropriate. A story he told about palliative care illustrates the point. A Russian prisoner of war dying from advanced tuberculosis was screaming in pain. Cochrane diagnosed pleurisy and administered analgesics, but to no avail. He wrote: "I felt desperate, and finally instinctively sat down in the bed and took him in my arms, and the screaming stopped almost at once. It was a wonderful education about the care of the dying". Cochrane wrote his own obituary, published in the BMJ after he died in 1988, and the last sentence read: "He was a man with severe porphyria who smoked too much and was without consolation of a wife, a religious belief or a merit award – but he didn't do so badly".

FURTHER READING

Anaemia

Turner A R. Haematological aspects (chap 9.14) in Doyle D, Hanks GWC, MacDonald N, Oxford textbook of palliative medicine 2nd Ed 1998. Oxford University Press.

Analgesics

Gannon C. The use of methadone in the care of the dying. European Journal Palliative Care; 1997; 4(5): 152–8.

Anger

Faukner A, Maguire P, Regnard C. Dealing with Anger in a patient or relative: a flow diagram. Palliative Medicine 1994; 8: 51–57.

Anxiety

Torben Bendix. The Anxious Patient 1982. Churchill Livingstone.

Ascites

Regnard C, Mannix K. Management of asites in advanced cancer – a flow diagram. Pallitative Medicine 1989; 4: 45–47.

Assessment

Maguire P, Faulkner A, Regnard C. Eliciting the current problems of the patient with cancer – a flow diagram. Palliative Medicine 1993; 7: 151–6.

Assumptions

Meystre CJN, Burley NMJ, Ahmedzai S. What investigations and procedures do patients in hospices want? Interview-based survey of patients and nurses. BMJ 1997; 315: 1202-3

Macbeth Pitkin R. Listen to the patient BMJ 1998; 316: 1252

Slevin ML, Stubbs L, Plant HJ et al. Attitudes to Chemotherapy: comparing views of patients with cancer with those of doctors, nurses and the general public. BMJ 1990; 300: 1458-60

Attitudes

Greer S, Watson M. Mental adjustment to cancer: its measurement and prognostic importance. 1987. Cancer Surveys; 6: 439–453

Audit

Berger A, Why doesn't audit work,BMJ 1998; 316: 875–6

Higginson I, Clinical Audit in Palliative Care, Oxford, Radcliffe Medical Press Ltd, 1993

Bereavement

Murray Parkes C, Coping with loss: Bereavement in adult life. BMJ 1988; 316: 856–9

FURTHER READING

Bleeding

Regnard C. Control of Bleeding in advanced cancer. Lancet 1991; 337: 974

Boredom

Lichter I, Mooney J, Boyd M. Biography as therapy. Palliative Medicine 1993; 7: 133–137.

Stevens E. Promoting self-worth in the terminally ill. European Journal of Palliative Care 1996; 3 (2): 60–64.

Breaking Bad News

Kaye P. Breaking Bad News – a 10 step Approach. 1995. EPL Publications.

Carers

Hannicq M. Family Care – new principles. European Journal of Palliative Care 1995; 2(1): 21–24.

Ramirez A, Addington Hall J, Richard M. ABC of Palliative Care – the carers. BMJ 1998; 316: 208–211.

Children

Knoll L, Barnes J, Jones AL, Stein A. Cancer in parents: telling children. Sensitive communication can reduce psychological problems.BMJ 1998; 316: 880

Black D. Bereavement in Childhood BMJ 1988; 316: 931–3

Sheldon F. Children and bereavement – what are the issues? European Journal of Pallaitive Care 1994.

Cognitive Therapy

Greer S. Moorey S. Adjuvant psychological therapy for cancer patiens. Palliative Medicine 1997; 11: 240–244

Aaron T. Beck, Cognitive Therapy and the emotional disorders. 1976 International Universities Press Inc.

Confusion

Stedeford A, Regnard C. Confusional States in Flow Diagrams in Advanced Cancer and other diseases. Edr Regnard C. Churchill Livingstone 1995.

Consent

Russon L. The implications of informed consent in palliative care. European Journal of Palliative Care 1997; 4(1): 29–31.

Constipation

Fallon M, O'Neill B. ABC of palliative care. Constipation and diarrhoea. BMJ 1997; 315: 1293–295

FURTHER READING

Consultation

Bryne PS, Long BEL, Doctor's talking to patients. A study of the verbal behaviour of GP's consulting in their surgeries. HMSO 1976

Neighbour R, The Inner Consultation: how to develop an effective and intuitive consultation style. MTP Press Ltd 1987.

Pendleton D, Schofield T, Tate P, Havelock P, The Consultation, a Approach to Learning and Teaching. Oxford University Press 1984.

Counselling

Mary Burton, Maggie Watson. Counselling People with Cancer. 1998. John Wiley and Son.

Gerard Egan. The skilled helper 1975 Brooks/Cole Publishing Company, California.

Counselling Couples

Stedeford A. Couples facing death – Unsatisfactory communication. A series of 2 articles in the BMJ 17 October 1987 (pages 1033–1036) and 24 October 1987 (pages 1098–1101) – both in volume 283.

Crowe M. The Treatment of Marital and Sexual Problems. Ch.13 In: Bentovin A et al, Family Therapy 1982

Crisis Intervention

Chung K. Brief social work intervention in the hospice setting: person-centered work and crisis intervention synthesised and distilled. Palliative Medicine. 1993; 7: 59–62.

Earnshaw-Smith E. We don't need to be God after all. Palliative Medicine. 1987; 1: 154–162.

Death Certification

Ashley J, Devis T. Death certification from the point of view of the epidemiologist. Pop Trends 1992; 67: 22–28

Decision Analysis

Thornton J G, Lilford R J. Johnson N. Decision analysis in medicine. British Medical Journal 1992; 304: 1099–1103.

Dowie J. "Evidence-based", "Cost-effective" and "preference-driven" medicine-decision analysis based medical decision making is the pre-requisite. J Health Serv Res Policy 1996; 1: 104–13.

Simes RJ. Treatment selection for cancer patients: application of statistical decision-making theory to the treatment of advanced ovarian cancer. J Chron Dis 1985, 38: 171–86.

Decision-making

Maher EJ, Goodman S, Jefferis A. Decision-making in the management of advanced cancer of the head and neck. Differences in perspective between doctors and patients: future avenues for research. Palliative Medicine 1990; 4: 185–189.

Dehydration

Ethical decision-making in palliative care: Artificial Hydration for people who are terminally ill. National Council for Hospice and Specialist Palliative Care Services 1997.

Denial

Maguire P, Faulkner A. How To Do It: Communicate with cancer patients: handling uncertainty, collusion and denial. BMJ 1988; 297: 972–4.

Depression

Tiernan E. Depression in Tuturiols in Palliative Medicine, Ed. Peter Kaye. 1997 EPL Publications.

Diarrhoea

Regnard C, Mannix K. The Control of Diarrhoea in advanced cancer – a flow diagram. Palliative Medicine. 1990; 4: 139–142.

Mercadantes S. Treatment of diarrhoea due to entercolic fistula with octreotide in a terminal cancer patient. Palliative Medicine. 1992; 6: 257–259.

Discharge planning

Stump N. Home assessment before discharge from a palliative care unit. European Journal of Palliative Care; 1994; 1(2): 96–7.

Wattess C. The benefits of home care for the terminally ill. European Journal of Palliative Care; 1997; 4(3): 90–92.

Hockley J. Rehabilitation in palliative care – are we asking the impossible? Pallaitive Medicinc. 1993; 7(suppl 1): 9–15

Dying

Murray Parkes C. Coping with loss: The dying adult. BMJ 1998; 316: 1313–5.

Bolund C. Loss, mourning and growth in the process of dying. Palliative Medicine 1993; 7(suppl 1): 17–25.

Manns-Bielders K. Saying goodbye. European Journal of Palliative Care. 1994; 2(1): 25–28.

FURTHER READING

Dysphagia

Wright RER, Jordan C. Videofluoroscopic evaluation of dysphagia in Motor Neurone disease with modified barium swallow. Palliative Medicine 1997; 11: 44–48

Lewis Jones CM, Sturgess R, Elershaw JE. Laser therapy in the palliation of dysphagia in oesophageal malignancy. Palliative Medicine 1995; 9: 327–330

Dyspnoea

Corner J et al Non-pharmacological interventions for breathlessness in lung cancer. Palliative Medicine 1996; 10: 299–305.

Booth S. The management of dyspnoea in advanced cancer. Hospital Medicine Hosp-med 1998; 59 (2: 98–99).

Boyd KJ, Kelly M. Oral Morphine as a symptomatic treatment of dyspnoea in patients with advanced cancer. Palliative Medicine 1997; 11: 277–281

Managing the experience of breathlessness 1996. The Institute of Cancer Research.

Emergencies

Falk S, Fallon M, ABC of Palliative Care. Emergencies. BMJ 1997; 315: 1525–1528

Ethical problems

Wilkinson J. The ethics if communication in palliative care. Palliative Medicine. 1991; 5: 130–137.

Evidence-based medicine

Rosenberg W, Donald A. Evidence-based medicine: an approach to clinical problem-solving. BMJ 1995; 301: 1122–6.

Sackett D L, et al. Evidence based Medicine: What it is and what it isn't. BMJ 1996; 312: 71–2.

Families

Smith N, Regnard C. Family Problems. In: Regard C, Hockley J Eds) Flow diagrams in advanced cancer and other disease, 1995, London: Edward Arnold

Cooklin AI. Family Therapy: Tenderness and toughness in the face of distress. Palliative Medicine 1989; 3: 89–95

Liossi C, Hatira P, Mystakidou K. The use of the genogram in palliative care Palliative Medicine 1997; 11: 455–461

Smith N. The impact of terminal illness on the family. Palliative Medicine. 1990; 4: 127–135.

FURTHER READING

Fentanyl

Yeo W et al. Transdermal fentanyl for severe cancer – related pain. Palliative Medicine 1997; 11: 233–239

Spencer I. Transdermal opioid control of cancer pain. European Journal of Palliative Care. 1996: 3(4): 147–149.

Ahmedzai S. Brooks D. Transdermal fentanyl versus sustained-release oral morphine in cancer pain: preference, efficacy, and quality of life. J Pain Symptom Manage 1997 May; 13 (5): 254–61.

Portenoy RK, Southam MA, Gupta SK, et al. Trans–dermal fentanyl for cancer pain. Repeated dose pharmacokinetics. Anesthesiology 1993; 78: 36–43

Genetic Counselling

Steel M. Cancer families and Cancer genes. Palliative Care Today. 1994. 3; 4–7.

Guidelines

Jackson R, Feder G. Guidlines for clinical guidelines. BMJ 1998; 317: 427-8

Grol R, et al. Attributes of clinical guidelines that influence use of guidelines in general practice: observational study. BMJ 1998 Sep 26; 317: 858–61,

Home Care

Doyle D. Domicillary palliative care. Oxford Textbook of Palliative Medicine 2nd Ed 1998, Oxford University Press.

Walters C. The benefits of home care for the terminally ill. European Journal of Palliative Care. 1997; 4(3): 90–92.

O'Niel B, Rodway A. ABC of Palliative Care in the Community. BMJ 1998; 316: 373–377.

Gomas J. Palliative Care at home: a reality or "mission impossible". Palliative Medicine 1993; 7(suppl 1): 45–59.

Information

Hibble A, Kanka D, Pencheon D, Pooles F. Guidelines in general practice: the new Tower of Babel? BMJ 1998; 317: 862–3

Muir Gray J A. Where's the chief knowledge officer? BMJ 1998; 317: 832

Judgement

Naylor C D. Grey Zones of clinical practice: some limits to evidence based medicine. Lancet 1995; 345: 840

FURTHER READING

Living Wills
Doyal L. Advanced Statements about Medical Treatment. Code of Practice. Report of the BMA 1995. BMJ Publishing Group

Lymphoedema
Todd J, Living with lymphoedema, Your guide to treatment, 1996, London: Marie Curie Cancer Care.

Morphine
Hank G W, et al. Morphine in cancer pain: modes of administration.BMJ 1996; 312: 823–6

O'Brien T et al. A randomized crossover trial study comparing the efficiency and tolerability of a novel once – daily morphine preparation (MXL capsule) with MST Continus tablets in cancer patients with severe pain. Palliative Medicine 1997; 11: 475–482

Mouth Problems
Kirkham S. Sore Mouth in Context. European Journal of Palliative Care supplement 2 (2)

Turner G. Oral Care for patients who are terminally ill. Nursing Standard, 1994: 8 (41): 49–54

Walls AWG, Murray ID. Dental Care of patients in a hospice. Palliative Medicine. 1993; 313–321

Nausea & Vomiting
Barnes M J. ABC of palliative care. Nausea, Vomiting and Intestinal distention. BMJ 1997; 315: 1148–1150

Nutrition
Taylor MC, Moran BJ, Jackson AA. Nutritional problems and care of patients with far-advanced disease. Palliative Medicine. 1989; 3: 31–38.

Rapin C. Nutrition for terminally ill elderly patients. European Journal of Palliative Care. 1994; 1: 84–87.

Boyd KJ, Beeken L. Tube feeding in palliative care: benefits and problems. Palliative Medicine. 1994; 8: 156–158.

Oncology decisions
Hoskin P, Makin W. Oncology for Palliative Medicine. 1998. Oxford University Press

Organ donation
Feuer D, Organ donation in palliative care. European Journal of Palliative Care, 1998; 5(1): 21–25

Callender S. Tissue Donation – an option after death. Palliative Care Today, 1998; Vol VII Number 11: 4–5

FURTHER READING

Pain

Hanks GW, Posteroy RK, MacDonald N, O'Neill WM. Difficult pain problems In Oxford textbook of Palliative Medicine (pages 257–274) 1993. Oxford University Press.

Sykes J, Johnson R, Hanks G W. ABC of Palliative Care, Difficult pain problems. BMJ 1997; 315: 867–869

Kearney M. Imagework in a case of intractable pain. Palliative Medicine. 1992; 6: 153–157.

Palliative Care

Emanuel E J, Emanuel L L. The promise of a good death. Lancet 1998; 351 (suppl II): 21–29.

Personality

Briggs Myers I, Briggs Myers PB, Gifts Differing (1980) Consulting Psychologists Press Inc, Palo Alto. ISBN 0-89106-011-01

Goldsmith M, Wharton M, Knowing me, knowing you – exploring personality type and temperament (1993) SPCK. ISBN 0-281-04652-2

This Myers-Briggs Personality Type Indicator (MBTI) was developed by Katherine Briggs, who was already developing her own classification of personality when she discovered Carl Jung's book of 1923 "Psychological Types". Briggs passed on her interest to her daughter, Isabel Myers, who was stirred by the sufferings of the Second World War to do something that might help people understand each other. So in 1942, with no formal training in psychology or statistics, Myers began to collect information. She analysed thousands of individuals on the basis of their preferences and developed the 4 scales to describe personality. The title of her last book "Gifts Differing" emphasises that it is in no way judgemental but all about differences.

Prescribing

Marinker M. Personal paper: Writing prescriptions is easy. BMJ 1997; 314:747–8

Drummond SH, Peterson GM, Galloway JG, Keep PA. National Survey of drug use in palliative care. Palliative Medicine 1996; 10: 119–124

Twycross RG, Bergl S, John S, Lewis K. Monitoring drug use in palliative care. Palliative Medicine 1994; 8: 137–143.

Pressure Sores

The prevention and treatment of pressure sores, Effective Health Care, October 1995 Vol 2, Number 1.

Problem-solving

Wood BC, Mynors-Wallis LM. Problem-solving therapy in palliative care. Palliative Medicine 1997; 11: 49–54

FURTHER READING

Research

Crombie I K. The Pocket Guide Critical Appraisal 1996. BMJ Publishing Group.

Wilkie P. Ethical issues in qualitative research in palliative care. Palliative Medicine 1997; 11: 321–324

Risk

Cook RJ, Sackett DL. The number needed to treat: a clinically useful measure of treatment effect. BMJ. 1995; 310: 452–4

Calman KC. Cancer: science and society and the communication of risk. BMJ 1996; 313: 799–802.

Barclay P, Costigan S, Davies M. Lottery can be used to show risk. BMJ 1998; 316: 1243.

Sleep

Eisen J, MacFarlane J, Shapiro C M . ABC of Sleep Disorders. Psychotropic drugs and sleep. Br Med J 1993; 306:1331–4.

Spinal Cord Compression

Hillier R, Bee Wee. Palliative Management of spinal cord compression. European Journal of Palliative Care, 1997; 4(6): 189–192

Spiritual Distress

Grey A. The Spiritual Complement of Palliative Care. Palliative Medicine 1994; 8: 215–221.

Cole R. Meditation in palliative care – a practical tool for self-management. Palliative Medicine 1997; 11: 411–413

Coates S. Spiritual components in palliative care 1995; 2(1): 37–39.

Steroids

Twycross R. The Risks and Benefits of Cortcosteroids In Advanced Cancer: Drug Safety 1994; 11(3): 163–178.

Focus on Corticosteriods CSM/MCA. Current Problems in Pharmocovigilance 1998; 24: 5–7

Stories

Hudson-Jones A. Literature and medicine: narrative ethics. Lancet 1997; 349: 1243–46.

Frank AW. The wounded storyteller: body, illness and ethics. University of Chicago Press, London 1995.

Brody H. "My story is broken; can you help me fix it? Medical Ethics and the join construction of narrative. Lit Med 1994; 13: 79–92.

FURTHER READING

Subcutaneous drugs

Bradley K. Swap data on drug compatibilities. Pharmacy in Practice; March 1996: 69–72.

Johnson J, Patterson S. Drugs used in combination in the syringe driver – a survey of hospice practice. Palliative Medicine 1992; 6: 125–130.

Terminal Phase

Changing gear – guidelines for managing the last days of life in adults. The National Council for Hospice & Palliative Care Services. 1997.

Lichter I, Hunt E . The Last 48 Hours of Life. Journal of Palliative Care 1990; 6: 7–15

Adam J. ABC of Palliative Care. The last 48 hours. BMJ 1997; 315: 1600–1603.

Back IN. Terminal restlessness in patient with advanced malignant disease. Palliative Medicine 1992; 6: 293–298.

Thinking

Denig P, Haaijer-Ruskamp FM. "Thinking aloud" as a method of analysing the treatment decisions of physicians" Eur J Pub Health 1994; 4: 55-59.

Transactional analysis

Thomas Harris. I'm OK – You're OK, 1967, Pan. Chapter 5. Analysing the Transaction.

Weakness

Gleeson C, Spencer D. Blood transfusion and its benefits in palliative care. Palliative Medicine 1995; 9: 307–313

Lichter I. Weakness in terminal illness. Palliative Medicine. 1990; 4: 73–80.

ABBREVIATIONS

AFP	Alpha feto-protein
BACUP	British Association for Cancer United Patients
BD	Twice a day
BRCA1	Breast Cancer Gene
BMJ	British Medical Journal
CA	Carcinoma antigen
CEA	Carcino-embryonic antigen
CLL	Chronic lymphatic leukaemia
CT	Computerized tomography
ECG	Electrocardiogram
ECT	Electro-convulsive therapy
ENT	Ear, Nose and Throat
FU	Fluorouracil (5FU)
G-I	Gastro-intestinal
GP	General Practitioner
h	hour
Hb	Haemoglobin
HCG	Human Chorionic Gonadotrophin
HIV	Human Immunodeficiency Virus
HT	Hydroxytryptamine (5HT)
ICP	Intracranial pressure
IM	Intramuscular
IV	Intravenous
JAMA	Journal of the American Medical Association
L	Litres (eg 5L)
L1	First lumba vertebra
MAOI	Monramine Oxidase inhibitor
MCV	Mean cell volume
MG	Milligram
MRC	Medical Research Council
MRI	Magnetic resonance imaging
MS	Multiple sclerosis
MST	Morphine sulphate tablet
MSU	Midstream Specimen of Urine

ABBREVIATIONS

NG	Nasogastric
NSAID	Non-steroidal anti-inflammatory drug
OD	Once daily
OGD	Oesophago-gastro-duodenoscopy
OT	Occupational therapy\therapist
PEG	Percutaneous endoscopic gastrostomy
PRN	Pro Re-Nata - when the need arises
PSA	Prostate specific antigen
P-V	Peritoneo-venous (shunt)
QID	Four times a day
QDS	Four times a day
RCT	Randonised Controlled Trial
RT	Radiotherapy
RTI	Respiratory Tract Infection
SC	Subcutaneous
SNRI	Serotonin and Nor-adrenaline re-uptake inhibitors
SSRI	Selective Serotonin re-uptake inhibitor
TB	Tuberculosis
TCA	Tricyclic anti-depressant
TDS	Three time a day
TENS	Transcutaneous electrical nerve stimulation
T4	Fourth thoracic vertebra
T10	Tenth thoracic vertebra
U & E	Urea and electrolytes
UCH	University College Hospital
U\S	Ultrasound
UTI	Urinary tract infection
WBC	White blood cell